BREAK OUT
OF YOUR
FAT
CELL

BREAK OUT OF YOUR FAT CELL

The Holistic Mind-Body Guide to Permanent Weight Loss

Jeane Eddy Westin

Foreword by: Jack LaPatra, Ph.D., author of
Healing, The Coming Revolution in Holistic Medicine

Published by

CompCare® publications

Minneapolis, Minnesota
A division of Comprehensive Care Corporation

(Ask for our catalog, 800/328-3330, toll free outside Minnesota
or 612/559-4800, Minnesota residents)

The author dedicates this book
to you, the reader, and to your
ultimate victory over the pain
of overweight

Other Books by Jeane Eddy Westin

The Thin Book, CompCare Publications

Finding Your Roots, Tarcher/St. Martin's

Making Do: How Women Survived the 30's, Follett

Contents

ACKNOWLEDGMENTS

No author ever writes a book alone. I had my encouragement and help from the following people to whom I offer my sincere appreciation: Dr. Trudy Helmlinger, who discussed the psychology of overeating and overweight behavior with me on numerous occasions; Delores Amlin, who led body-image workshops; William L. Asher, M.D., president of the American Society of Bariatric Physicians for his suggestions; Helen Sparks for her personal and proffessional expertise and to my family who remained loving and uncomplaining when meals were late and I rode my Exercycle during a favorite television program.

Special thanks are deserved by my editor Diane DuCharme and my agent Jane Jordan Browne who believed in this book.

Introduction

I rarely use the word "holism" any more. For several years, I conducted research on holistic health and finally wrote a book on the subject. During those efforts, the word "holism" was firmly embedded in nearly every sentence I uttered. In recent years, however, popularization of the term has so blurred its meaning that I've purged it from my vocabulary. Nowadays, healers of many persuasions claim they have been practicing holistic medicine all along. And masseurs even offer holistic massages. Jeane Westin and her book have made it possible for me to write about holism again.

The concept of holistic health is so wonderfully simple. It's only common sense to think of a human being in terms of the functions implied by the words — mind, body, spirit, and emotions. Most of us realize that these parts interact, and that an impact on one function will often influence the others. It follows then, that healing or adjusting one part must, of necessity, consider the other parts. That is exactly the approach that Jeane Westin's "holistic guide to weight control" takes.

I feel very strongly about the importance of each person making a "commitment" to his/her own health. Commitment means that a man or woman is willing to give high priority to health right along with family, work, recreation, and other important facets of a person's life. You begin with a foundation of knowledge and willingness to learn, add intense self-awareness, and follow with a plan for the division of your life force between mind, body, spirit, and emotions in a way that the condition of concern receives healing energy in a holistic manner. The previous sentence describes, in a nutshell, Jeane Westin's conceptual approach to weight control.

The ideas of holistic health have been around for a long time, but a specific strategy for the use of the ideas to solve a personal problem such as overweight has never been better illustrated than in this work. The reading of this book was a holistic experience for me, and I know it will be for you.

Jack LaPatra
(Author of *Healing, The Coming
Revolution in Holistic Medicine*,
McGraw-Hill, 1978)
Atlanta, Georgia

BREAK OUT OF YOUR FAT CELL

The Holistic Mind-Body Guide
to Permanent Weight Loss
by
Jeane Eddy Westin

Whether you are young or old, rich or middle class, black or white, single or married — if you're overweight — you can learn coping techniques to help you live a whole and satisfying life *while you take pounds off.*

Break Out of Your Fat Cell begins where most "diet" books (and doctor visits) have ended, just as you're starting a period of calorie deprivation and emotional conflict. Here is a book to take with you every step of the way, a book from which to learn and a book which will confirm that you have every right to the body and life you want.

It is obvious to most of us that overweight people need more, much more, than they're getting. Most dieters today need a release from guilt and an identification with others in the same boat. They need strategies to win against the pressures placed on them by a thin chauvinistic society; and above all, they need to develop a new sense of self-worth — an attitude which demands that the world treat them with respect.

Until now, there have been few sources, outside of expensive therapy or general self-actualizing books, to give the overweight the practical, non-dietary help they need to build their deflated self-esteem so that they can diet successfully. Instead, dieters face a continuous barrage of ego-deflating propaganda from thin America which implies: "You are not sexually attractive, not employable, uninsurable, and lack the moral equipment (will power) to push yourself away from the table." All this while the media blitzes them with high-calorie food advertising.

The attitude toward overweight in our society can be perceived as a Catch-22, huckstered as we are to eat more than we need, and then programmed to self-loathing over the result.

Diets alone, even the best medically supervised ones, have not been entirely successful. According to the National Council on Obesity, the overweight population has increased 450 percent in the past decade, a decade marked by more dieting than any other in our history. The latest Gallup Poll further indicates that now 60 percent of all adult Americans consider themselves overweight.

What else can be done that is not now being done? The intriguing concepts of holistic medicine, with its emphasis on a *total* mind, body, spirit approach to "wellness," seem to hold an important answer for overweight people. In this book, you will learn how to apply this concept to your weight problem and your life.

I believe *Break Out of Your Fat Cell* will offer you the non-condemnatory, self-assertive, self-actualizing way to live you have been looking for while you diet off unwanted pounds. It seems obvious that a dieter who listens to his or her own voice, has self-respect and demands respect from others, will be more successful at dieting than one who is anxious, self-lascerating and easily manipulated.

Nevertheless, this book does not assume a "fat power" stance. There seems to be no such utopia (at least in America) where fat can be beautiful. But neither is overweight ugly, sinful, disgusting, or unsexy. It is a living problem which requires utilizing every possible resource to solve — and that's all.

This book says to you: Sure, you want to diet so you'll be happier and healthier, but to be permanently successful you can, indeed *must*, live a full life while you're losing weight. Isn't that a message you have been waiting to hear?

Break Out of Your Fat Cell will help you do just what the title says. As you read, you will build self-esteem so that you can begin to· lose weight, continue to lose weight or maintain a hard-won weight loss — permanently. I hope each chapter will lift more of the burden of guilt and self-blame from your shoulders so you can at last go to work for yourself, a self that you truly love.

As you reduce your guilt and increase your cope-ability you will come to this simple truth: "I am a wonderful human being just the way I am, but I want to find a way to be even better."

You have probably read dozens of pro-diet books. Now get ready to read your first pro-dieter's book.

Sacramento, California

Living well is the best revenge.
— *Gerald Murphy*

Chapter One

Stop Blaming Yourself

First things first: forget about every diet that ever failed, about every eating binge you've ever had, about every exercise plan that didn't work, about every broken vow you've made to yourself. Those failures have nothing to do with you today.

Next, stop blaming yourself for being the bad person you *think* you are. Nobody likes to talk about it, but in this "thin is everything" society fat people are supposed to be lazy, dumb, ugly, asexual, sleepy, sloppy, passive, gluttonous and clownish. Only a real oaf would label us so to our faces, but on an unconscious level even the kindest, most sensitive people can harbor this prejudice. Worst of all, and on that same unconscious level, we overweights have been brainwashed to feel this way about ourselves, and feeling this way, many of us accept half a life as our just due.

Can you believe it? Along with the burden of excess pounds we carry around a built-in prejudice, hating ourselves, buying every mean and petty thing said by fools.

Enough! It is about time we overweights stopped participating in our own degradation. Maybe we can't change today's thin-oriented culture (most of us wouldn't want to), but we certainly can change the way we think about ourselves. Throw away the old negative labels. They are only excess baggage.

This time you are going to win at the weight-losing game. Why? Because this time you will have a whole body plan that recognizes what a wonderful person you *already* are, a plan that lets you live and work and socialize, a mind-body plan that will help you break out of your fat cell.

Don't doubt your ability to turn your life around. What's that? You've heard you have no will power. Who says? Living fat in a society that makes a virtue of thinness and a sin of fatness requires extraordinary strength of will. The problem is to direct that strength in a totally new way.

Spend a little of your strength right now to understand why you are overweight in the first place. You have been told that overweight is caused by eating too much, eating the wrong foods and getting too little exercise. That is true, as far as it goes, but it doesn't go far enough. This book presents some exciting new scientific thinking on the problem which may cause you to question the validity of blaming yourself for being fat. Now if you didn't blame yourself so much, you might begin to feel better about the person you are, and feeling better, be able to do more to help yourself lose the pounds you want to lose — permanently. What could possibly be wrong with that? Read on.

You're Not Too Fat, Just Too Late — by 25,000 Years

Go back now beyond your known genealogy to a time when your distant ancestors, clothed in animal skins against the glacial cold, sat huddled in shallow caves. One day your grandfather, 10,000 times removed, takes his primitive weapons to the ice's edge and makes a big kill on which his family feasts ravenously. They have gone for days, perhaps weeks, without anything to eat but a few seeds scraped from under the snow and a burrowing animal or two your ancient grandmother caught in her snare.

Why is this scene important to you in the Twentieth Century?

"Man's prehistory in Europe, Russia and northern China," says physical anthropologist Anne Scott Beller, "is that of a species making its way at the edge of a glacier whose unpredictable stops and starts had a direct and sometimes cataclysmic effect on the prevailing food supply.

"Survival therefore dictated some metabolic compromise between feast and famine, and *the emerging species must have survived through the ability of those who could store food under their own skin* and live off this store until climate or hunting renewed their larder." (The italics are mine.)

Beller in her marvelous book *Fat & Thin: A Natural History of Obesity* concludes that survival was nature's reward for those who could store the greatest amount of fat and release it as frugally as possible. Is it any wonder that even present-day populations still contain large numbers of people whose genes dispose them to overweight?

Dr. Abraham Weinberg, a New York psychiatrist, goes further and says that our minds as well as our bodies cause overweight in the twentieth century. "It's due to a folk memory," Weinberg says, "of the days when we used our bodies instead of our refrigerators

2

to store food. Fat meant staying alive and, deep down, our brain still remembers."

There you have a unique new look at the problem of why people get fat. Buried not too deeply in our unconscious is the memory of starvation along with fat genes coded for survival at any cost. But does this mean we are victims of our ancestry, condemned to fatness when we no longer need it to exist? Of course not. We can't allow these ancestral genes to dictate obesity down through the milleniums any more than we can let them send us an urge to hit our mate over the head with a club.

What we can and must learn from these ancestors of ours is that our tendency to gain weight has to do, in part, with our genetic makeup and not our moral character.

Do these scientific theories mean we are not to blame for our overweight? Yes, that is exactly what they mean. However, that doesn't absolve us from taking responsibility for controlling the fat-storing ability that we no longer need.

Overeating: a Survival Reflex We Can't Use

The problem, as Beller and so many others have pointed out, is that times have changed and changed drastically. What was once a lifesaving tendency to store fat and stay alive long after the thinner members of the tribe starved to death may today be life-threatening, at least according to many medical doctors and insurance actuarial tables.

The fact is, we no longer have a food supply problem. Instead of feasting occasionally and starving the rest of the time, most of us eat three very square meals a day. That old genetic urge to store against the coming ice age, not due for another 20,000 years or so, is playing havoc with our bodies and lives today.

The Earth Mother Legacy

Overweight, especially in children, has been popularly supposed to be just another rotten thing your mother did to you — stuffing and overfeeding you into early blimphood. For many of us, this stereotype is exaggerated. If we want to blame mother, we must look beyond our biological mom to our prehistorical Earth Mother.

This will come as a complete surprise to most overweights (especially women), but by the time human beings marched into the New Stone Age (these are the ancestors we've been talking

3

about), they worshipped life-giving corpulence in the image of an Earth Mother goddess. These ample stone Venuses have been found from France to Siberia and were immortalized by ancient sculptors because of their magnificent fat deposits.

Although we have discarded our ancestors' sense of deity, the next time your diet-deflated fat cells send your mouth "eat-eat" messages, don't blame yourself, blame it on a nagging Earth Mother.

One question remains: Do we get fat because we eat too much, or do we eat too much because we are programmed to store fat? The evidence suggests that an abundant food supply coupled with a drastic decrease in physical activity combine to produce a lifestyle for which nature did not design our bodies. The argument may go on for years to come, but at least now you should be totally unwilling to allow anyone to wave an old moralistic finger in your face. And for heaven's sake stop blaming yourself. If you need more convincing, read on.

The Cardinal Sin Factor

Eating, as columnist Ellen Goodman has observed, has become the last bonafide sin. Because we live in an era when people recognize that alcoholism/drug addiction is a disease and that lack of opportunity contributes to criminal behavior, all of society's disgust can now be focused on highly visible overweights. We are not judged and do not judge ourselves for who we are or what we do, but for our size. If we are pounds over the prevailing thin ideal, we have "sinned" in the ancient sense of that word. We even use the language formerly reserved for religious transgressions to describe our behavior. We say, "I was really *tempted* to eat that dessert," or "The *devil* made me eat that." Even those newly liberated masses who find sex such a joy look on a roll of fat as immoral.

The result of this modern dietary morality is that overweights see themselves as bad and thin people as good. Nothing could be less true.

"Obesity is not a sin," says Dr. Jean Mayer, the highly respected nutritionist. "At most, it is the consequence of errors of omission, the result of not having kept up the lifelong battle against an environment which combines constant exposure to food with the removal of any need to work for it physically."

It's bad enough that overweight fills us with self-loathing; it also empties our pocketbook in subtle ways. "Some fat people pay a penalty of $1000 a pound," reports Robert Half, head of a top personnel agency. Another executive recruitment firm states flatly that obesity damages careers. They found that excess weight could cost an executive $10,000 a year in salary. How can this happen? A number of factors are at work. Part of the loss is due to prejudice against the overweight being accepted by the so-called prestige colleges in the first place, then by employers who won't promote the overweight and finally by overweights themselves who quit halfway up the ladder of success. But the main factor, as you can guess, is simply image. Personnel directors want to hire slim, good-looking people. Oh, how we pay and pay for the "sin" of being fat!

Remember, all this discrimination continues while our culture carries on an open love affair with food. There is an essential ambivalence (psychiatrist Theodore Rubin calls it schizophrenia), nowhere more visible than when magazine diet articles have four-color food ad displays on facing pages. The strong message overweights get over and over again is "Eat, but don't get fat."

The anti-fat mania has gone far enough, at least as far as fat people are concerned. We can't change the minds and hearts of the "big-ots" overnight, but we must change our self-blaming attitudes about ourselves so that we can get on with the task of losing weight for a healthier life.

It is well known that many of the victims of Nazi oppression came to identify with their oppressors, and viewed themselves with the same contempt that their concentration camp guards did. We overweights, ill-treated and discriminated against, in the past have agreed with our oppressors. No more! We must reject the Puritan heritage that regards overweight as sinful, that makes us feel inferior to thin people. Nothing saps the energy we need to lose weight and live a whole, healing lifestyle faster than a pervasive feeling of guilt.

But oppression is not overcome by a pious hope that it ought not to be. It is overcome by action. Take these steps today and every day.

1. Love yourself and allow yourself to experience all the things you want to do with your life.

2. Don't accept this culture's concept that you are a gluttonous, immoral being because you are overweight.

3. Stop feeling inferior because of your size and concentrate on the things you do well.

4. Decide to lose weight because you *are* a wonderful person, not in order to be one.

If you take nothing else away from this chapter, take this: NOBODY EVER GOT FAT BY BEING BAD; NOBODY EVER GOT THIN BY BEING GOOD.

Morality has absolutely nothing to do with losing weight. The right diet coupled with proper energy expenditure plus lifelong perseverance and integration of your mind and body — that's the permanent weight loss equation.

The Cardinal Sin Factor is dead. Bury it. For good. For your good.

No-fault Dieting

There is a new way of tackling big problems which has become increasingly popular in the last few years. It is called the no-fault principle. Whether the term refers to auto accidents, divorce or doctor's malpractice insurance, no-fault means that no one is held to blame for what happens to go wrong. It is about time we overweights applied no-fault to dieting.

We can't begin to truly get rid of our overwhelming guilt, the guilt that is keeping us fat, until we stop blaming ourselves for every dietary lapse. No one, fat or thin, eats exactly what he or she should every day. (So why are you blaming yourself for what is only average behavior?)

The trick is to have enough self-esteem to give yourself all the chances to get thin you will ever need, day after day. Don't fall into the trap of fearing failure to the point that it prevents you from giving yourself another chance to win.

As I said in *The Thin Book,* tell yourself that "nobody's perfect" and really mean it. Expecting perfection of yourself is an intolerable burden. It requires you to be unkind, impatient and intolerant with yourself, the very self-incriminating attitudes you will find least helpful if your goal is permanent weight loss.

Specific diets are seldom our problem. Most nutritionally sound diets result in weight loss. Searching for the one "magic" diet is usually just a way of postponing serious confrontation with life change. After all, who knows more about diets than fat people? No one.

Perhaps the most important ingredient in no-fault dieting is not the ratio of protein to fat to carbohydrate, but how you view yourself as a whole person. Are you willing to make mistakes, pick yourself up and go ahead in the sure knowledge that you are a wonderful human being? If you can apply the no-fault principle to your diet, as well as to your automobile, then you are on your way to constructive and permanent change.

Eliminate "Fat Thinking" to Make Your Diet Work

No matter how frustrated and full of self-blame you have been in the past, take the stance from this day forward that life is for you and not against you. When we overweights expect the worst, that is usually what we attract. When we have a healthy self-concept that liberates us from negative "fat-thinking," we can learn to accept, and even love, ourselves, while at the same time losing weight.

"The paradox is that we must accept ourselves as we are," says psychiatrist Theodore Rubin, "if we want to change ourselves." The doctor doesn't mean that you don't have faults, things you want to improve. What he does mean is that as long as you define yourself in terms of size, worthlessness and blame, you have a poor chance of dieting successfully.

You are a good person. Eliminate negative "fat thinking" that drags you down to defeat. Accept yourself and love yourself. That's the difference between living with your mind separated from your body and living whole. Author Ralph Trine says: "Thoughts are forces; like builds like, and like attracts like. For one to govern his thinking, then, is to determine his life."

Hang on to that idea. It is a lifesaver if you are determined to think and live positively.

Dieting Plus: the Mind/Body, Holistic Approach to Permanent Weight Loss

How many diets have you tried? If you're like many of us who have been fat all our lives, (or even just for a short time) you have tried them all — no fat, low fat, high protein, low carbohydrate, grapefruit, booze, water and even the nothing (fasting) diet. Perhaps you have dreamed up some exotic diets all your own. Did they work? Probably. At least for a time. But they didn't work permanently because our problem is not hunger. Sure, you are hungry, maybe hungrier than thin people because of your response to external cues. We will talk more about your marvelous appetites (that's right, they can be a positive force) later. The fact is that dieting alone has not solved the weight problem of 80 MILLION fat people. Why? Let's look at the new "holistic health" revolution for our answer.

7

Diets haven't worked for us and that doesn't make sense. Or does it? Holistic medicine tells us that not dieting alone, but a host of factors in our daily lives influence our ability to lose weight and keep it off. This "new medicine," as it is sometimes called, preaches that an individual has to deal with his or her whole person, all aspects of body, mind and life, not just with the part causing the problem.

You don't need to become a medical expert in order to practice holistic health, also known as "positive wellness." What you need is to become an expert on your own body. Here is where you *must* stop blaming yourself for past diet failures. The more you tune in and accept your body, the better you are able to take care of it in a way that will promote mind-body integration. The more you know your body — its feelings, its symptoms, its real appearance — the better you can take charge of your life and start losing weight for good.

This new weight losing concept is nothing more nor less than a lifestyle assault on obesity.

Dieting alone is like applying a Band-Aid after brain surgery and sending the patient home to take his chances. The mind-body holistic approach cares for the total person and promotes completeness in everyday living.

Don't doubt for a moment that there can be a close relationship between body and mind. Holistic health expert, Dr. Jack LaPatra, suggests making a few simple observations which will show you just how integrated they really can be.

1. How do you walk when your spirits are high or low?
2. What are your eye movements when you feel uncomfortable?
3. Do you have a special odor on a bad day?
4. Is your touch light or heavy when you are unsettled?

You can probably think of many other ways in which your mind and body work together. Ask yourself why they cannot work together to lose weight. The answer must be that they can.

That is what *Break Out of Your Fat Cell* is all about. Coming chapters will deal with your mind and body in a number of unique ways. You will gain special insight into what is known about obesity and that super "baddie" white sugar; next you will learn how to demand respect and get it; then you will find out whether or not fat people are sexy. (Here's a hint: WOW!) Finally, you will

8

discover how to find the best doctor and diet group for your personality, how to win the battle against the biggest sabotage effort since World War II, how to cope with weight problems in your own children, and last, a survival kit of "goodies" to complete the new you.

It is no secret why all of these chapters come after this one on self-blame. If you continue harassing yourself, you become your own worst enemy. Remember: YOU ARE NOT TO BLAME. This concept is the bedrock of a successful holistic weight control program. Sure, people are prejudiced against overweights (as sometimes we are against ourselves) and it is true that you may be genetically predisposed to store fat, but that does not mean you are doomed to be fat all your life. You can take charge of your life today, you can cope with overweight and you can learn to live in the fullest most enjoyable sense of the word.

Somewhere down the road you are going to be 10 pounds or 50 pounds or even 100 pounds lighter, but today love yourself for what you are, as you are, so that you make change possible. Make the most of your mind and body. Don't dress as if you are attending a funeral, or lower your head in shame. You have nothing of which to be ashamed. Why, the mere idea is simply ridiculous!

A Short History of Dieting
from Classical Age to Space Age

Hippocrates issued the first medical warning against obesity in 450 B.C. He wrote that the fat "are more likely to die suddenly than the slender." Nevertheless, the Venus de Milo was not all that skinny, proving the Greeks were no more able than we to follow their doctor's diet advice. One explanation for the overripe Venus comes from Dr. Jean Tremolieres, director of the Laboratory of Human Nutrition, Bichat Hospital, Paris. He believes that in times when mankind feared starvation, fat women were beautiful. "Men were reassured by a woman's plumpness," he says, "that their fear of starvation would not come true."

By the first century, the Romans had already developed the modern ambivalence of talking diet and eating with high-calorie abandon. "A well-governed appetite is a great part of liberty," decreed Seneca, who concentrated on the body. "Reason should direct and appetite should obey," coaxed Cicero, who concentrated on the mind. But while these sages were delivering their aphorisms, wealthy Romans ate reclining on couches while slaves passed among them with bowls and feathers so they could regurgitate to eat again — and again.

Even the Dark Ages shed some light on the continuing human problem of dieting to avoid obesity. In the eleventh century, the French were ruled by a monarch known as Louis the Fat. Royal physicians bled the King as a diet aid without much success. His precise dimensions are not recorded, but his subjects called him "the bruiser."

At about the same time, the church, in the person of St. Jerome, was railing against its fat monks. The venerable saint issued this memorable put-down of monks who didn't lose weight. "A fat paunch," he sniffed, "never breeds fine thoughts."

During the sixteenth century reign of England's Henry VIII, the king became so fat that special machinery was required to transport him from one part of his castle to another. There is no record that the king's physicians ever suggested he diet or in any

10

way commented negatively about his avoirdupois, since Henry had an unfriendly way of taking your head off when displeased.

This age was also a period of full employment for full-blown artist's models. Leonardo da Vinci, Michelangelo, Raphael, and Rubens all painted women whose fleshy abundance would repel today's fashion photographers.

Only one of these old masters gave the weight of his subjects another thought. Leonardo, during the years he worked on the Mona Lisa, also took time to invent the self-indicating scale. The next time you face the "white monster" in your doctor's office blame it on Leonardo.

"Whoever heard of fat men heading a riot?" asked Washington Irving, no lightweight himself. " 'Tis your lean, hungry men who are continually worrying society . . ." In this case, Irving had not done his homework. Even a cursory glance at pictures of our founding, and very revolutionary, fathers shows a number wearing considerable paunches. Revisionist historians even believe George Washington's likeness was deliberately slenderized by patriotic painters who put the great man on a diet he was never on himself.

Until the nineteenth century, obesity was generally a problem of the affluent. But the Earth Mother's long dormant fat cells were just waiting to break out in the general population. The Industrial Revolution gave them their chance. As the middle class grew, so did its weight problem.

By 1900, dieting was such a concern that some young Americans went so far as to swallow "sanitized" tape worms in order to lose weight. But the modern diet craze really began in the 1920's when women wanted to make their figures "boyish" to fit into stylish flapper clothes.

The arrival of the space age brought with it a galaxy of diets, nutritional data, obesity research and behavior modification. More attention is focused on overweight than on any other single health problem on the planet.

The Hunger Mystery

Do you find yourself hungry all the time and feeling guilty about it? Here are a couple of reasons why the hunger, but not the guilt, is perfectly natural.

Life first appeared on the earth in the form of single-celled creatures which were, very simply, eating machines. From this beginning, the Earth Mother implanted in all her children an instinct we call self-preservation. This instinct is primarily concerned with feeding the body so that it may be kept healthy.

The need of human beings for food and drink is so basic that nature rewards its fulfillment with immense pleasure. To be hungry, on the other hand, brings instant discomfort. It is obvious that nature provided this pleasure-pain mechanism to keep us alive.

Early in our history, there developed dual aspects to our striving for food. In one instance, we tried to control nature by growing our own crops, to enlarge and ensure the source of our food supply. In the other instance, we began a struggle to control our own nature, our compulsive need to satisfy the hunger of the moment without regard to depletion of food supply, or in modern times, weight gain. The reason behind this behavior is that nature makes the pangs of immediate hunger inescapable, and the consciousness of tomorrow's hunger remote. Some cellular memory goads us on to eat and drink for tomorrow we may die.

Later in our history, food and God became inextricably entangled. Like Erysichthon in Greek mythology, who was cursed by the Gods with an insatiable appetite until he finally devoured himself, we can risk divine disapproval if we succumb to physical appetite. No one knows at what point along the eons that driving hunger force within ceased to be simply biological and became, through increasing awareness, a longing to be as one with the Spirit. Out of early rituals to find God, we began to partake of food offerings to the gods, not to satisfy our physical hunger but to satisfy our spiritual need to hold a closer communion with God. With such a human history, it is no wonder that today we know hunger as both an urgent reality and an inexplainable mystery.

HOLISTIC LIFESTYLE CHANGE 1

Make a list of all the things for which you blame yourself. Take a week or more so you will have a good collection. Then complete this exercise to discover the many aspects of self-blame in your life and to decide what to do about them.

Blame Balance Sheet

I blame myself for	This is absurd because	A positive feeling would be
1.		
2.		
3.		
4.		
5.		

Chapter Two

Understanding Your Weight Problem

Why me? At some time in your overweight career you have flung this question heavenward, not expecting an answer perhaps but not understanding why there wasn't one either. As you grew older, and hopefully wiser, it soon became clear that overweight was not merely a sadistic whim of the gods but the interaction of a number of diverse forces. In this chapter, we will take a look at many of them, how they affect you and finally, what you can do about them.

To begin with, any plan of attack against a major living problem must include programming your mind with as much information as you can find.

It is impossible to feel guilty or live your life in self-blame if you have enough knowledge.

You don't have to go back to school and squeeze behind one of those little desks to learn more about overweight. Here is a brief overview which will give you a deeper insight into your problem.

Overweight America

A recent Gallup poll asked a cross section of men and women whether or not they were overweight. Sixty percent answered yes. They were young and old, educated and uneducated, wealthy and broke; they represented all religions, races and ethnic groups. Clearly, overweight in the modern world is an equal-opportunity problem. No matter where you fit into that 60 percent "minority," you are obviously not alone. The Earth Mother had many children.

Whatever your personal degree of overweight, it is a small amount considering the size of the total problem. It has been calculated that there are five BILLION extra pounds being carried around by fat Americans for which they pay $10 BILLION a year — not to maintain them but to get rid of them. Even accounting for deflated dollars and inflated prices, that is a hefty sum to pay for a diet answer that has, so far, eluded many. And we will go on paying, according to a market study by Frost & Sullivan which showed the diet industry growing at a rate of 20 percent every year with no end in sight. There are now so many diet products, machines and over-the-counter aids for sale that both San Francisco and New York City have lately held Diet Expos, the latter in Madison Square Garden, scene of countless other heavyweight encounters.

The diet industry isn't all sell. Most of the nitty-gritty work is done by the dieter, at home, alone. It has been estimated that 308 million diets are started in this country every year. There are no estimates on how many are successful. Those statistics are shrouded in agonized silence.

The interest in diet reaches to the august floor of the United States Senate. In 1977, the Select Committee on Nutrition and Human Needs issued a 79-page report calling for major changes in eating habits. Loaded with scientific testimony, the Committee's goals call for a sharp reduction in the amounts of cholesterol, fat and sugar in the average diet, and a sharp increase in the consumption of fruits, vegetables and fiber. Here is how experts say we should apportion our daily nutritional intake:

Fat	30% (10% saturated, 20% unsaturated)
Protein	12%
Carbohydrate	58% (43% complex, 15% sugar)

Of course, nutritional experts, like all experts, don't agree completely, but the universal message comes through loud and clear. The average American diet, which currently accounts for almost half its calories in fat and another one-fourth in sugar, is sadly out of balance. Based on these figures it doesn't take an expert to agree that everyone's diet needs an overhaul. How is your food intake divided nutritionally? What changes would you like to make?

If you are ready to feel *guilty* because your diet is deficient, don't fall into that trap just yet. Consider the hostile environment in which you live. Everywhere there are Coke and candy machines. Television bombards you with advertisements for sweet snacks. A charming voice sings, "Canada Dry tastes like love," and a happy family demonstrates that "Nothing says lovin' like something from the oven." Is it any wonder that so many overweights, yearning for love, have problems dieting when the media temptress warbles the Earth Mother's siren song?

What have you learned so far about your weight problem?

1. The majority of Americans are overweight, and this includes people from all walks of life.

2. Many are dieting with limited success and paying a great deal of money for the privilege.

16

3. Even though we are eating so much, while one-third of the world is starving, we are eating poorly, a diet composed of too much fat and sugar.

4. Overweights live in an environment which emphasizes food, particularly high-calorie snack food.

All this could be discouraging, but it need not be. Knowing these facts gives you added ammunition to succeed. Such knowledge illuminates the problems of being fat in America and puts us on our guard. Sometimes just recognizing a situation that affects us helps us to do something about it. Recognition is a big part of the solution — recognition without guilt.

Meanwhile, the search for the "cure" for fat has led overweights to a plethora of faddish diets, clinics, devices, shots, pills and consciousness-raising sessions. We have tried a hundred and one methods, first working on the body, then on the mind. No method has totally succeeded, because the body and mind do not work separately. Defying geometry, the holistic dieter knows that the whole person is *more* than the sum of its interacting parts. The mind and body acting *together* can accomplish what never could be done by the mind and body at a distance from each other.

What Is Meant by the Terms Overweight and Obese?

The medical community has a standard guide they use to determine who is overweight and who should be classed as obese. There are slight variations but these percentages are the rule of thumb:

Overweight = 10 percent over natural body weight
Obese   = 20 percent over natural body weight

The magazine *Medical Opinion* recently estimated at least 66 million (or the majority of too-heavy Americans) fall into the obese category. That means if you are too heavy, you are more likely to be obese than overweight. For the overeater, the chances of being a little overweight are about as good as being a little pregnant.

What Causes Overweight?

You know by now that you are not isolated in the problem of overweight. Just the opposite; you have plenty of company. You also have an array of possible causes which you should know about so that you can take action appropriate to your whole body. Dr. A.D. Jonas, a New York psychiatrist, says "There are as many reasons for obesity as there are fat people." These reasons can be genetic, sexual, environmental, metabolic and psychological. Get acquainted with the causes you think might apply to you.

Science doesn't know everything about the causes of obesity. It is known that increased energy consumption in the form of calories and decreased energy expenditure causes obesity. But why it causes obesity in some people and merely overweight in others, and why some obese maintain their fat while others lose on the same calorie count is still a mystery.

It seems obvious that there is a predisposition to accumulate fat that can only be regarded as genetic, so let's look at that factor first.

The Genetic Factor

To deny the influence of fat genetic heredity, when over 1,500 physical and mental conditions can be traced to a genetic chain, is an arrogance the strictest social moralist would not attempt.

Even though statues of the Earth Mother have been discovered over a wide area of the world, the genetic factor in obesity might be underestimated even today were it not for a classic bit of research with twins.

In 1937, Dr. H.H. Newman showed that identical twins who always have identical genetic characteristics weighed approximately the same in adulthood while fraternal twins who do not have the same genetic makeup varied by as much as 50 percent. Other confirming studies have shown that identical twins raised in separated environments ended up very close in weight.

If you had one fat parent, your chances of being fat, too, are about 40 percent, but if you had two fat parents and got a double dose of fat genes, your chances of gaining too much weight are better than 80 percent.

Remember, the *ability* to gain extra and unnecessary weight need not be realized, due to other precautions you can take. The genetic factor only means you have potential for fat, but this fat trait will not manifest itself unless other factors are present as well, such as overeating and underexercising.

Part of the genetic factor in overweight has to do with body types. Dr. William Sheldon was the first to divide human bodies into three basic types:

1. Ectomorphs are long, slender "Twiggy" types who can eat whatever they like and never put on a pound.

18

2. Mesomorphs are usually muscular, square solid types who can have a weight problem if they overeat or stop their usual high level of physical activity.

3. Endomorphs are a familiar body type for overweights. They have a rounded shape, are short-limbed and "hippy." Endomorphs can gain excess weight, it is said, by merely passing close to a chocolate eclair.

Which do you think is your body type?

The Sex Factor

Dr. Barbara Edelstein, author of the not-to-be-missed *Woman Doctor's Diet Book for Women,* has documented the role gender plays in obesity. "There is no escaping the fact," she says, "that we were ordained as baby receptacles, so nature has seen to it that we will never be without fat." She explains that it doesn't matter whether women actually bear children; nature pads them anyway, just in case.

Other studies confirm the doctor's diagnosis. "The average man has a body fat content of 14 percent compared to 25 percent in the average woman."

Another aspect of the sex factor is hormonal. Testosterone, the male hormone, helps a man to lose fat, according to some experts, at twice the rate a woman loses. On the other hand, female estrogens and progesterones are naturally fat-producing and fat-hoarding. Even the synthetic hormones present in birth control pills have the same propensity. It seems that nature doesn't care whether hormones are natural or synthetic; it uses both to make a woman fatter than a man and to keep her that way.

The Environmental Factor

Every new bit of information you put into your mind tears a hole in the thin fabric of self-blame and guilt. Now let's peek through another hole and learn more about the hostile environment in which most fat people in America live, an environment that behaviorists tell us is loaded with cues that stimulate us to eat and overeat. Research makes it clear that most overweights are extremely sensitive to:

1. Food that is easily obtained. We don't like inconvenience, so modern convenience foods, or "fast-foods" are right down our alley.

2. Television come-ons and brightly colored food ads.

3. Food attractively displayed in so many places we can hardly avoid contact unless we become hermits.

Another component of the environmental factor in obesity is social, which includes ethnic and cultural tendencies. Most every overweight knows someone who took lessons from Portnoy's mother, someone (not necessarily a woman) who forces food as an expression of love, hospitality or cultural compatibility. This excess no longer takes place exclusively in the home, since 43 percent of the work force is now female. "I have worked in offices," says one desperate dieter, "where women came to work with homemade blintzes, tacos and potato pancakes. But the worst offender was a man who passed out hot slices of fresh sesame-wheat bread he'd popped out of the oven in the wee hours before work."

The final element which makes the environmental factor so potent in the fight against overweight is one of economics. Costs of high-grade protein, especially meat, spiral ever upward, leaving our plates to be filled too often with less expensive starchy carbohydrates. It is no wonder that statistics show a rise in obesity as real income drops.

The Metabolic-Endocrine Factor

It has been years since most of us have heard — "I have a glandular problem." This statement has been held up to so much ridicule in the past few decades that very few overweights say it today, even though new evidence suggests that it can be, at least in part, true.

Our bodies are like metabolic combustion engines, highly complex and multi-functional. One person can eat or exercise with more efficiency than another. The caloric energy you use climbing stairs can vary greatly from the energy expended by your thinner colleague. Given the variables, it is impossible to state categorically that the obese do not have "glandular problems," although doctors don't know whether they are induced by obesity or vice versa.

Dr. Neil Solomon, author of several books on obesity and weight reduction, put this chicken-or-egg controversy in perspective: "A possible explanation (for the up and down in weight Yo-Yo syndrome) is that an important metabolic capacity is weakened or exhausted while the patient is overeating. Then when he cuts back his caloric intake his body is unable to metabolize certain foods properly.... At the moment, we do not know whether a particular case of obesity begins with a weakness in the hormonal-enzymatic apparatus or whether obesity induces the weakness."

A lengthy parade of metabolic factors plays a role in whether or not you gain too much weight in the first place, and how fast you can lose it. An underactive thyroid gland, a lack of pituitary hormones, an upset in female or male hormones, hyperactive adrenal glands, faulty insulin production and elevated blood fats are only a few of the metabolic and biochemical factors that can create a potential weight gain problem. Your doctor should check for all of these possibilities, or refer you to an endocrinologist.

Some weight experts believe that the so-called "appestat," a device in our brain that tells us when we are hungry, may have been set too high in some of us, accounting for the reason we eat far too much for body health maintenance.

Depending on an individual's metabolic mix, investigators have found that it can take as little as 1,250 to as much as 3,000 calories to add a pound of fat to a patient's weight. That is a variation of close to 250 percent! This could be one explanation why some people lose weight at such a slow rate, and some never gain too much to begin with. No wonder we begin to suspect, after years of denial, that we may very well have "gland" problems that scientists haven't even discovered yet.

The Psychological Factor

For most of this century, the overweight have been defined as psychologically sick, using the old Freudian model of the neurotic, mouth-greedy, adult baby. One of the most hopeful signs today is that obesity is no longer treated as a mental sickness by many psychiatrists. Psychoanalyst Theodore Rubin, who once said all overweights were sick, no longer believes this to be true. "Ordinarily overweight people," says Dr. Rubin, "are no sicker psychologically than thin people."

We may even be a bit saner. Fat people as a group have less schizophrenia and only just as much psychoneurosis as thin people do. Other studies in England have shown that city-dwelling obese are more stable than urban thin people.

That is not to say that we overweights don't suffer psychologically from the results of society's oppression and, in some cases, need to seek out psychological treatment. (This is discussed in more depth in Chapter Eight.) Some very common emotional problems asociated with obesity and emotional overeating are anger, boredom, hostility, frustration, helplessness and a sense of failure. These seem to be fairly reasonable emotional problems considering what we have to contend with on a daily basis, although they may cause more severe coping problems that will require professional help.

It is interesting to note that less and less is heard about obesity as a mental sickness since intestinal bypass surgery for the massively overweight created an opportunity for scientists to measure emotional health after drastic and sudden weight loss. In the past, we overweights have been warned that our underlying psychological problems would be with us even after we lost weight, and that we had better care for them before dieting or, at the very least, concurrently.

Here is what the Dartmouth Department of Psychiatry reported to the National Institute of Mental Health after a recent study of bypass patients who had lost dramatic amounts of weight:

> The general response to weight loss was an improvement in mood, self-esteem and interpersonal and vocational effectiveness, body image and activity levels. The most significant psychological change responsible for improved functioning seemed to be the loss of a pervasive sense of entrapment associated with obesity. The reversibility with weight loss of many of the psychosocial disturbances associated with severe obesity supports the view that they are *as much a consequence as a cause of excessive adiposity.* (My italics.)

Of course, this does not mean that some overweights do not have mental problems. They do, just like their thin friends. What it does mean is that we are not fat because we are crazy. And for some of us who have spent a lifetime questioning our sanity, this can be the most liberating news of all.

These are a few arguments which show the overweights are influenced by many factors. The great truth is that obesity in modern humans is so many-faceted, that if it is to be solved, it must be attacked simultaneously from many angles.

Cures, Now and Future

If a safe, inexpensive sure cure for overweight were announced tomorrow, the line of customers would stretch halfway around the world. Unfortunately that day is not in sight, but here are some interesting possibilities either being tested or proposed in theory. None is on the market.

1. **Glycerol:** Why do you eat too much? Two University of Illinois researchers, Psychologists John Davis and David Wirtshafter, believe that the blood level of glycerol, a natural component of fat tissue, may turn the body's desire for food on and off by acting on special cell receptors in the brain. Experiments on animals have shown that glycerol significantly lowered weight by dramatically reducing food intake. Davis and Wirtshafter believe that glycerol acts on cells in the hypothalamus, which they think switch on the appetite when glycerol levels in the blood fall and turn it off when they rise as a result of eating. Although overweights have a chronically high level of glycerol circulating in their blood already, their appetite cells may have stopped responding to fluctuations in the substance. Conceivably, glycerol injections might override this defect and cause weight loss as it did in laboratory animals. More testing needs to be done.

2. **Perfluoroctyl bromide:** This drug which could "make diets obsolete" has been reported by three University of Illinois pharmacists. Again laboratory animals (one suspects there are a great number of svelte rats running around laboratories) were fed this drug which is said to coat the lining of the stomach and intestines to prevent food from being absorbed into the blood stream. PB, which acts as a barrier, causes food to pass out of the body rather than become deposited as fat. The Food and Drug Administration has not approved the drug for use.

3. **Fake Fudge:** Here is a way to have your future cake and eat it too. Obesity expert, Dr. George Bray of the UCLA School of Medicine, is working with a food firm which plans to manufacture cookies, candy, cakes, bread, ice cream — all the dieter's forbidden fruit — but make them indigestible so they pass through your system without adding many calories. They smell, look, feel and taste like sweets, but again, an FDA go-ahead is needed before the product can be marketed.

4. **Fat Antibody:** Here is more evidence that the old gland alibi may not be an alibi after all. Acting on a hunch, Dr. Irving Perlstein of the University of Louisville ran some special blood tests on overweights with normal thyroid tests. In a significant number of patients, he discovered that although their bodies produced the thyroid hormone, some organs released an antibody that neutralized it. It was as though the thyroid gland wasn't working at all, even though the standard thyroid tests indicated everything to be normal. When these patients

were given daily doses of synthetic hormone carefully measured to suppress the neutralizing antibodies, they showed a dramatic weight loss. No one knows how many overweights have antibodies which set up barriers for their body's own thyroid hormone, but Dr. Perlstein urged fellow doctors to do more studies and not to be so quick to shrug off overweight as simply a case of overeating. "Obesity is a complicated metabolic disorder," he says, "which presents itself in many forms."

5. Kidney Bean Cure: Dr. John J. Marshall, a University of Miami biochemist, has discovered a protein in the uncooked kidney bean that appears to inhibit the body's utilization of glucose. Called phaseolamin, the substance sprinkled on food caused laboratory animals to absorb fewer calories. The substance has not been used on human subjects since raw kidney beans contain toxins harmful to people.

Most of the "cures" now under investigation are passive in nature in that they do not require an exercise of mental will to lose weight. You take a pill or sprinkle a powder or get a shot. Other research on laboratory animals, which surgically inflicts lesions on the hypothalamus for weight loss, raises questions of *Clockwork Orange* or *1984*. So-called fat liberationists theorize that in a society that abhors fat, such mind control could be forced on the overweight, regardless of their own wishes in the matter. These overweights claim they have a right to be fat if they desire.

The only current "cure" offered by medical science to the obese is bypass surgery. This high-risk operation (only brain surgery is riskier) consists of shortening the intestinal tract from its normal eighteen-foot length to a short eighteen inches. As a result, fewer calories (also fewer vitamins and minerals) can be absorbed by the body and the person loses weight. Quite often an enormous amount of weight is lost, especially in younger patients, but a significant number of people do stop losing while still much too fat.

Just like everyone else, post-bypass patients have to watch their diet. They can't consume too much fat, sugar or alcohol in any form because their liver might not be able to handle these foods. Liver failure is the most feared aftereffect of the surgery and can lead to another operation to hook the intestine back up again. Other aftereffects are lifelong diarrhea, vitamin deficiencies and other potential health problems such as gall stones and kidney stones.

Very few of us are candidates for such a drastic solution to obesity. Surgeons generally have a criteria that patients must:

1. Be more than 100 pounds over (some even require double) their natural weight.

2. Have failed in every other diet method for at least five years.

3. Be a person whose life is endangered by obesity.

4. Be a good psychological risk, that is a person who is emotionally stable and can comply with years of follow-up care. Emotional stability is usually determined by a psychiatrist's evaluation.

This surgery is very expensive and can take as long as four to five hours on the operating table, so that patients, despite their excess weight, have to be fairly good surgical risks. Doctors estimate that only about five percent of all overweights qualify for bypass surgery.

From this chapter, you have learned that obesity is not the outcome of a single determining factor, but of many complex factors. We have explored these complex factors of why we get fat and for just one reason: to give you knowledge, and out of that knowledge, reduce your guilt.

"Guilt is the number one problem with the obese person," says bariatrician (weight specialist) Peter Lindner, M.D. "It is probably the most destructive state of mind for any weight control program and is also responsible for some of the emotional overeating that takes place. Resulting irrational thoughts and ideas and incorrect interpretations lead to even more overeating."

Though you have every right not to feel guilty about being overweight, you must still take responsibility for improving your life, and that means your health. People get fat because they overeat, and they stay fat because they overeat. It's true you may have genetic, environmental, metabolic and psychological predispositions to be overweight — some of these, or even all of these — but the bottom line is just this: you have a potential for overweight that does not have to be realized or can be reversed if you take responsibility for your health right now.

YOU ARE NOT A GLUTTON. You have a physiological or psychological tendency to put on more pounds than you need for living in this era of food abundance. You also have the intelligence (as we'll see later, maybe more than your thin brothers) to tap deep levels of power within yourself and restore harmony to your whole person.

You have a powerful enemy in your desire to overeat, but you have an even more powerful ally in your mind and body. Use them to help you take control of your own life. Here are four take-charge steps you will want to get started on.

1. *Determine what factors influence your overeating.*

Ask yourself what environmental, cultural or other variables cause you to eat too much.

2. *Determine how these influences can be overcome.*

One example might be deliberately choosing foods that do not reinforce an ethnic eating pattern.

3. *Identify the effects of overeating that you don't like.*

Take a good look at your life and remember that obesity takes the fun and adventure out of it. It makes you huff and puff and fear social occasions where you probably have more to offer than many thins.

4. *Develop a plan to gain control of your whole person.*

A part of this plan may require you to drastically change your lifestyle. Be open to new dieting and living experiences. Assume responsibility for your own perpetual wellness by finding ways to use your mind-body power to lose weight.

Taking charge is a complex performance which cannot be developed all at once. We overweights have thought of ourselves as fat slobs for so long that it may take some time to think through to a dignified personal regimen for weight loss and life change. Simply telling ourselves to change is not enough. We must perform these new behaviors and reinforce these new attitudes so often that they become potent forces in our lives.

Change is possible! By consistently eating wisely and well, you are constantly reaffirming your ability to take charge of your life. The connection between self-control and self-esteem has been observed since classical Greek times and is no less true today. Perhaps it is not enough to tell yourself to stop feeling so guilty about your weight problem; you may actually have to gain some small measure of eating control in order to end the process of guilt and self-blame. Haven't you noticed how a sense of order in one area can serve as a model in another? Remember, in school, once you had learned Spanish, it was much easier to learn French. The same principle works here.

Change is even more possible when we overweights become the masters, rather than the victims, of our potential for fat. The idea is to assert yourself, put yourself in charge of your whole person.

You have already taken two giant steps out of your fat-padded cell. One, you deny self-blame and refuse to degrade yourself. Two, you are armed with an arsenal of information and have an awareness of the problems of overweight which will help you build your commitment to life-change. You must realize by now that the most creative use you can make of your life is to make good use of yourself and what you are here and now.

In the next chapter, we will look at the single, most powerful stumbling block to successful dieting, weight loss and the good life — and how to whip it once and for all.

The First Diet Book

A *Letter on Corpulence* by William Banting, published in England in 1863, has the honor of being the first of a very long line of books about dieting. The story goes that Banting, a London undertaker with a stomach so huge he had to back down stairs, had been desperate to lose weight just a year prior to writing his book. Consulting a surgeon named William Harvey in a time when sweating, vinegar and all sorts of less than miraculous cures were current, Banting was ordered to cut down on sweets and starches, a daring and innovative prescription for that day and not bad advice even now.

This is exactly what Banting did. He omitted plum puddings, cream cakes and potatoes from his diet and one year later, according to his book, he had lost 46 pounds and along with them his huge stomach. Out of this experience, the enthusiastic Banting published his *Letter* to help others in their fight against "corpulence."

HOLISTIC LIFESTYLE CHANGE 2

1. Decide which factor(s) influences your weight problem most and by what percentage:
   Genetic
   Sexual
   Environmental
   Metabolic
   Psychological
2. What can you do to bring each factor under better control in your life?
3. Return to the list of things for which you blamed yourself at the end of Chapter One. Which ones have fallen away?
4. Read one informative book about obesity such as *Fat & Thin: A Natural History of Obesity* by Anne Scott Beller.

Chapter Three

Crime in the Sweets

We live in a sugarcoated society. From the cradle to the grave, from baby formula to pot-luck dinners at the senior citizens' home, sugar is a big part of our lives — and for some of us a big part of our bodies.

There are few overweights who are not hooked on sugar in some form. No one gets fat from eating rutabagas. Oh, some say they never eat candy or cake, but if you take a good look at their diet you will find sugar hidden away in the cereal, bologna and ketchup they eat. Most of us who became fat as children have known from a very early age that our "sweet tooth" is helping pile on the pounds. What we don't know and aren't told is that sugar can make us sick, nearly ruin our lives.

I wasn't always hooked on sugar. When I was about four years old and on an outing with my aunt, an elderly gentleman, who thought he was doing me a kindness, gave me a piece of white candy. Thinking it was soap, I took it home to my mother who was persuaded that I was old enough to eat it. She hadn't let me have candy heretofore, afraid I would choke on it. Needless to say, I didn't choke. It slid down with the greatest of ease, this first of very many pieces of candy and every other manner of sweet known to man. In later years, when I was 100 pounds overweight, the oldsters loved to recount the story of "when Jeane didn't know what candy was" at family gatherings.

As I grew into fat, pimply adolescence, my love for sugar in any form took a criminal turn. For one whole year, I withheld my church offering and exchanged it for secret butterscotch sundaes at the neighborhood soda fountain. That same Christmas, I ate most of the family's holiday cookies my mother had baked in advance, disguising the almost empty containers with rolled-up newspapers.

My extreme love of sweets made a sneak of me. After my family stopped being amused at my prodigious appetite for goodies and started to search for ways to discourage me, I became, literally, a "closet sugarholic." During the rest of my growing-up time at home, I ate my pints of ice cream, whole cakes and pies in the linen closet, or when the weather was nice, on the fire escape three stories above the street. It obviously never occurred to me that passersby below might think it strange to see me dangling from a ladder fifty feet above the street surrounded by a ledge full of home-baked pastries.

For most young people, adulthood may hold fantasies of exotic places, high-paying jobs and fancy cars, but for me, it meant two other, quite different, things. I discovered that by living alone, I could eat whatever, and whenever, I wanted, without bringing down disapproval on my head, and that I could save money by doing my own baking. Within a short time my expertise with the oven rivaled that of a Cordon Bleu pastry chef.

That is not to say that I didn't go on periodic diets and lose prodigious amounts of weight by cutting out sugar and cutting down on other carbohydrates. After one of these slim-down episodes, I married and, in a replay of what is now a familiar story to you, began to gain back my lost weight — and once again found myself hiding with my sweets in the closet, this time hiding from my husband. I remember wondering during one of these escapades if I would be standing in a closet stuffing down cookies when I was eighty years old!

Over the years, I gradually added to my weight problem an array of ailments which hung on even after I permanently lost 100 pounds. At first, I didn't tie them to my sugar habit, because I was eating so much less sugar than I had ever eaten before. What I didn't know was that I had gradually built up a physical intolerance to refined sugar that caused me to have violent physical and emotional reactions whenever I ingested even moderate amounts.

Intolerable migraine-like headaches, sleepiness, hangover symptoms, nausea, uncontrollable and unexplainable weeping spells and a brain that felt like mush by midday were, I assumed, my lot in life. Now, as a professional writer with assignments and deadlines, it is impossible for me to tell a grumpy editor, "I'm sorry, boss, but I couldn't get that story in on time because I was having a sugar blackout."

I don't know where I first got the message that sugar did more to me than just make me fat. I didn't get that news from doctors, who talked about moderation and prescribed Valium for my symptoms. It was a gradual awakening until the day I fully realized that sweet, sticky, syrupy sugar had invaded every corner of my life. I was hooked. I was addicted to junk food and the only way out was to kick it cold turkey just like any other junkie.

Within seventy-two hours (it takes about three days to get the junk out of your system), I felt younger than I had for years and had more energy than I could ever recall. I no longer needed to nap every afternoon, my headaches disappeared, my tears dried up and I immediately lost seven pounds of bloat. Sugar had acted on my body like salt acts on other bodies, binding water and causing me to swell uncomfortably toward evening. I felt like a new woman, one who had been given a new lease on both body and mind.

How Does White Sugar Work in the Body?

For maximum mind-body efficiency the amount of glucose in your blood must balance with the amount of blood oxygen. When everything is working well, this balance is maintained with fine-tuned precision by your adrenal glands. When you take refined sugar (sucrose or $C_{12}H_{22}O_{11}$), it is just a step away from being glucose so it escapes most chemical processing in your body. The sugar goes straight to the intestines, there to become glucose. This, in turn, is absorbed into the blood where your glucose level is already in precise balance with oxygen. What happens? The glucose level in your blood is thus drastically increased. Your delicate balance is destroyed and your body is thrown into crisis from glucose overload.

Somewhere in your brain an EMERGENCY light flashes on. Hormones pour from the adrenal glands and marshal every chemical resource for dealing with sugar, including a clarion call for insulin from the pancreas. Sometimes your body goes too fast and too far, the bottom drops out of your blood glucose level and you're in a second crisis right back where you started, needing some energy quickly.

After years of this, the body and brain can just give up, worn out with the continual backlash of producing too many hormones. According to William Dufty in his definitive and highly readable book *Sugar Blues*: "This disturbed function, out of balance, is reflected all around the endocrine circuit. The brain may soon have trouble telling the unreal from the real; we're likely to go off half cocked. When stress comes our way, we go to pieces because we no longer have a healthy endocrine system to cope with it."

After decades of being fat, working with fat people and writing about obesity, I'm aware that suggesting to anyone that they divorce refined sugar and marry abstinence from it, not just for the duration of a diet, but forever, is tantamount to asking for a place high on their "hit" list. Maybe you are able to eat sugar in moderation and then stop, with no physical or emotional side effects. If you can, my hat's off to you. But if you suspect you have a problem with sugar, then this chapter may help you identify and solve this problem. You will be armed with facts which will help you form a take-charge attitude about your whole body. That's how we break out of our fat cells.

A Land of "Sugarholics"

When our Pilgrim ancestors settled in North America, they consumed a bare four pounds of sugar a year. By the time of the Civil War, this figure had risen to 25 pounds a year, and now over a century later, Americans are eating about 125 pounds of refined sugar and syrups every year. This means that one out of every four calories you eat every day is without any nutritional value at all. One wonders if today's sugar-soaked Americans could have settled a new land, walked across a continent or protected an emerging nation with a Snickers bar and a Coke for sustenance.

If we were only just a little softer as a people, there might not be too much cause for concern. After all, we can fly across the continent today and we don't have too many fields to clear or log cabins to build. But being "soft" isn't the whole problem. The increased consumption of what has been called "white gold" has led to a number of health problems we must be concerned about.

Everyone knows or should know that increased sugar consumption and diabetes seem to go hand in hand. Between 1965 and 1973, diabetes increased more than 50 percent, affecting more than 5 percent of the total population. At this rate (6 percent increase every year), the number of diabetics will double by 1988. The average American has better than a one in five chance of developing the disease and double that chance for every 20 percent he or she weighs over the normal scale.

If you don't like those odds, you will like these even less. If you have a sweet tooth, the only thing you are likely to get from it is fillings. You stand better than a nine in ten chance of having a mouth full of cavities or, like 20 million other American adults, losing half your teeth.

32

Sugar is no sweetheart for your heart, either. Dr. John Yudkin, emeritus professor of nutrition at London University, heads a growing body of scientists who link a high-sugar diet with coronary heart disease. He has a mass of statistics covering diet and heart disease from all over the world, from which he concludes that there is at least as much evidence against sugar as against saturated fat.

And that's not all. There is evidence implicating a lot of sugar in the diet with high blood pressure, kidney stones, allergies, gout and dyspepsia.

Last of all, but not least of all, sugar is the big fat nothing — no nutrients, only calories — with which we Americans eat ourselves into obesity, and no one has to tell you what a problem that can be.

As much as most of us overweights like our sugar, you will be surprised to learn that we consume only 24 percent of it in confections. The other 76 percent is eaten when we don't even know it. If you can't believe these figures, the next time you go to the supermarket, read the labels on seemingly unsweet cans of soup, vegetables, mayonnaise, peanut butter, baked beans, chili, ketchup and mustard — yes, even mustard! While you're at it, check the ingredients on bread, bouillon cubes, dinner rolls, bologna, pastrami, yogurt and cereals. Get the picture? Eliminating or cutting down on sugar is going to take a great deal of determination on your part.

Most of us are aware that there are a great many chemical food additives today, but few of us would consider sugar a harmful additive. Perhaps we should. It may be the most harmful additive of all for fat people.

Refined sugar in food is just this: an additive, a sweetener, a cheap filler, a texturizer and a preservative. It does not make us stronger or give us the only source of quick energy. In fact, because of its effect on blood-sugar levels which you read about earlier in this chapter, it may do just the opposite.

174,600 Empty Calories Every Year

What does all this sugar mean in terms of pounds of fat? Our sugar intake must be seen in this context: at four calories per gram, the average 125 pounds of sugar per person per year, means we now consume 500 sugar calories a day. That is the energy equivalent of more than *50 pounds* of weight gain a year! Considering that most overweights do not fall into the average con-

33

sumption category (you know if you don't), it is hard to tell how many pounds of fat that means to each one of us.

If we overweights cut out or reduced our intake of refined sugar, it's obvious we would lose weight, provided we maintained our other food consumption and energy expenditure at the same level. We would reduce our chances of becoming diabetic by half and we would be less likely to get a long list of possibly damaging health problems. Yudkin, the high priest of low-sugar diets writes in his book *Sweet and Dangerous:* "If only a small fraction of what is already known about the effects of sugar were to be revealed in relation to any other material, that material would promptly be banned."

Sugar, it's clear, makes us fat and unhealthy. Then why don't we stop eating it?

The Unknown Addiction

Although there is no scientific data to substantiate the theory of sugar addiction, more and more scientists are considering the possibility. Dr. Sanford Siegal in his book *Natural Foods and Permanent Weight Loss Diet* says emphatically, "I believe sugar is addictive." He adds that he has no scientific proof but he thinks seventeen years in practice observing sugar-eating patients must be worth something. "The overindulgence in sugar consumption is unbelievable," he goes on. "There are patients who tell me that they don't stop eating until they vomit. In my own case I've noted that it's the first piece of candy that's fatal . . . once I have the first piece, it's almost impossible to stop."

One recovered "sugarholic" and later a board member of Overeaters Anonymous is convinced sugar can be as addictive as alcohol. After years of sharing the experiences of other OA members, she has concluded that "many of us use sugar like a drug. It is our lover, friend, comforter, and when stress comes into our lives we reach for it automatically. Giving it up is terribly difficult; many people go through withdrawal and get the shakes. For some of us, complete abstinence is the only way out. We cannot be social sugar eaters just the way other people cannot be social drinkers."

Psychologists have suggested that the "addictive personality" is prevalent in this era of instant gratification. Dr. Mehl McDowell of the UCLA School of Medicine, for one, reports that, thankfully, the addictive behavior of "sugarholics" disappears entirely *when sugar is eliminated from the diet.*

The Hypoglycemia Connection

It is impossible to leave the subject of sugar addiction without following the hypoglycemia connection to its end. Hypoglycemia or hyperinsulinism or low blood sugar — three names for the same condition — is the other side of the coin from diabetes. It is also much more prevalent, the estimates ranging upwards of 22 million American sufferers.

In hypoglycemia the ducts in the pancreas are oversensitive to sugar. When we eat something sweet, the pancreas pushes out too much insulin, causing our blood sugar level to drop. People with hypoglycemia are always hungry and they have other interesting symptoms as well: headache miseries, tension, exhaustion, anxiety and a heart that races and skips around until you're frightened you're having a heart attack.

Legions of hypoglycemics, mostly obese women, troop to their doctor's or psychiatrist's office seeking relief. Until recently, most were told "it's all in your mind." Now many physicians are beginning to use the six hour glucose tolerance test (GTT) to pinpoint any abnormal ups and downs in body glucose levels. Indeed, some mental health experts are suggesting a GTT test before anyone submits to psychiatric counseling. The symptoms of hypoglycemia are sometimes so emotionally severe that patients can assume they have mental problems.

What's the cure? "There is no glamorous cure that can be bought in a package," says one doctor cited in A.W. Pezet's *Body, Mind & Sugar.* The only sure cure is to kick sugar — refined sugar.

Remembering the hostile environment we obese live in (as you read in Chapter Two) you may ask, "How *can* I kick the sugar habit?" You're on to the sugared, chocolated and frosted media blitz or you wouldn't even ask that question. Awareness is half the solution.

Recognizing Media "Sweet Talk"

Our ancestors, if they were lucky, sometimes stumbled across a hive of wild honey, but that was the limit of prehistoric goodies until about 2,500 years ago when someone (no friend of ours) discovered a way to produce a crude sort of sugar by drying the sap of sugar cane. Although this unfortunate invention probably originated in India, some early PR flack banged the drums so loudly that it was not long before the invention spread to other parts of the world.

Today, the food industry is banging those same drums with an annual advertising budget which approaches FIVE BILLION dollars, a great proportion of it going to push heavily sugared, highly salted and fat-saturated snack foods. Nutritionist Dr. Jean Mayer recently pointed out that these "modified" foods now comprise over 55 percent of our total intake as compared to only 10 percent in pre-television 1941. Mayer believes that this increased consumption is the direct result of saturation advertising in the television sugarland.

The foods you grew up eating and liking are usually the foods you continue to eat and enjoy. If you grew up eating sugary, salty and fat-saturated foods, you will continue to eat them, much to the delight of the Earth Mother's waiting cells. Advertisers, knowing this, sweet talk you as often as six times an hour into buying goodies. Don't think it is only kids who are influenced. You are, too.

The Boston based group Action for Children's Television (ACT) says television creates "a strong desire for sugary foods which commercials inspire." Even anti-sugar parental guidance is not able to counteract the pervasive, corrosive influence of TV. One reason could be that for every dollar the food industry spends on junk food commercials, it spends two cents on nutritional education. There is some doubt that we even get our two cents' worth.

Don't think there is something wrong with you if you like sugar. "Man has a natural liking for sweet things," says Dr. Yudkin, "and a firm belief that foods that are palatable are good for them."

This love of sweets and its concurrent rationalization might not have been too harmful when we were satisfying ourselves with an occasional finger in the honey while the bees had their backs turned. But today, sugar is so pervasive in so many of our foods that it begins to resemble alcohol and tobacco. It is a material for which people rapidly develop a craving, while having no bodily need for it at all.

This is not a chicken-or-the-egg controversy. Human beings already have a well-developed liking for sweets, but the taste makers, by playing on this natural affinity, have turned a pleasure into a nightmare for our overweight society.

Every overweight man and woman should heed the ancient consumer warning: *Caveat emptor.* Beware of foods you buy and how much sugar in any form they contain. (Watch for listings of dextrose, corn syrup and sucrose, too.) Don't assume that a food has no sugar in it until you have read the label and assured yourself that sugar is not listed above the fourth or fifth ingredient. If it is, then the product probably has too much sugar for anyone on a weight-losing diet. It certainly has too much sugar for anyone who has decided that life could be oh so much sweeter without it.

How To Live Sugar-Free for a Thinner, Healthier Body

The inevitable question is: Where do you go from here? As in all lifestyle decisions, the choice is really up to you. You may decide that you don't need or want to eliminate man-made sugar from your life entirely. If so, you can take steps to cut your sugar consumption while getting the sweetness you crave. For example:

1. If you take two spoons of sugar in your coffee, cut the amount in half.

2. If you don't like diet sodas, try mixing half regular soda with half diet soda for a reduction in sugar intake.

3. Always use a non-sweet mixer for liquor.

4. You can look for the less sweet variety of desserts such as pound cake or go totally sophisticated and European and have cheese and fruit after a meal.

Try to get your refined sugar consumption down to about twenty grams a day, roughly based on this chart.

Sugar content of food and drink

1 level teaspoon of sugar	5 grams
1 bottle regular cola	12 grams
1 8-oz glass fruit drink	20 grams
1 teaspoon of jelly	5 grams
1 2-oz piece of cake	10 grams
1 4-oz piece of fruit pie	20 grams
2 squares chocolate bar	30 grams
1 oz candy	20 grams
1 scoop ice cream	12 grams

It might be fun, or maybe not, to determine how many grams of sugar you have eaten today. Do you think you can live with 20 grams or the equivalent of two cups of coffee with two teaspoons of sugar in each? If the answer is no, then maybe you should rethink your decision to reduce but not eliminate sugar for good. You may be more hooked than you know.

Dr. Yudkin recommends a gradual tapering-off, just eating a little less sugar every day until you have it down to a saner level. Many overweights, including myself, have not been successful trying to just eat less. Most of us have to quit cold, eliminate as much sugar from our diets as the sugar-soaked food industry will allow.

Does that mean you will never, ever again, be able to savour the sensuous sweet? Of course not. There are clever ways to fool your taste buds while doing a wonderful thing for the rest of your mind and body.

Getting Your Just Deserts

Now that you're through being a sugar junkie, here's a recipe for the sweet life. First you blend a little daring with a generous scoop of imagination, add some quality foods and mix with a dash of determination for a dish which will help you stay slimmer, healthier and mentally sharper. Every meal you eat will be sweet revenge.

What can you do when you feel a sugar attack coming on? Try these sweet deceivers:

1. Eat a sour pickle or even some sauerkraut. You will be surprised how the salt-sour taste satisfies a craving for sweets.

2. Crunch on celery or chopped lettuce, both of which leave a sweet, clean taste in the mouth.

3. Have a piece of fresh fruit. It is full of nature's own sugar.

4. Drink a diet soda; it is sweet-tasting and filling. (Watch out for bloat with any carbonated beverage.)

5. Have some coffee with a dash of cinnamon or a glass of tea with fresh mint for sweet variety.

6. Whip some fresh fruit of the season with chilled, skimmed milk for a natural "shake."

7. If you are really desperate, try some of the dietetic candies, but watch out for hexitol, sorbitol and manitol, all high calorie chemical sweeteners contained in most varieties.

8. Dufty, in his *Sugar Blues*, advocates a great substitute for chewing gum — buckwheat lettuce you can grow yourself. "Chew it," he says, "and you'll be astonished at the natural sweetness."

9. For a tasty nibbler, try dried fruit you've dried yourself in one of the new, inexpensive food dryers. These foods open up a whole new range of sweet sensations and, again, they are very chewy.

10. If you must sweeten something you are cooking at home, use a *small* amount of honey or molasses. The operative word here is small.

11. If you are a chocolate addict, you can turn a chocolate diet soda and some powdered skim milk into a chocolate milkshake.

12. Try pouring unsweetened fruit juice over another fresh fruit for a super dessert. For a real taste treat add a *drop* of Marsala wine.

13. Buy unflavored, unsweetened yogurt and add your own fresh fruit and artificial sweetener.

14. Use natural sweeteners (if you're diabetic check with your doctor) such as honey, which takes up to four hours to metabolize; blackstrap molasses, which has 30 times more nutrients than cane sugar and maple syrup which is a rich source of potassium and calcium. Nutritionally, all these natural sweets are better for you than sugar, but for dieting they are still high in calories, so take it easy. Other naturals you may want to consider in small quantities are carob powder, carob syrup, sorghum syrup, date syrup, date sugar and barley malt extract.

15. Watch for other "natural" and no-calorie sweeteners being developed to replace cyclamates and saccharin. One substance is hesperidin made from citrus fruits; others are coming from a small red African berry and the common artichoke.

You will be amazed after only a few days of sugar-free living to discover that your body wants you to eat this way. When you have really become used to taking very little or no sugar in your food and drink, you will begin to notice that all your foods have a fantasic range of interesting flavors which you had hidden under the overwhelming taste of sugar. You will find out you had forgotten or never knew how good food could taste. You may even discover, although you'll never believe it now, that you begin to lose your desire for sugary foods. This Buddhist saying so well fits the thesis of this chapter:

> If you look for sweetness
> Your search will be endless
> You will never be satisfied;
> But if you seek the *true* taste
> You will find what you are looking for.

Sugar poses a threat to the national health, and even more to the point, to your own health. What are you going to do? If you're overweight, you probably have trouble with refined sugar in some degree already. Now is the time to make a decision, take control of your life, take charge of your body and mind.

Let go of any belief system based on helplessness, hopelessness or self-blame. The holistic attitude toward health is that you have the power to heal yourself. No one else can do it for you, or do it better than you can. If you have made your decision about the sugar in your life, then you are ready to go on and assert yourself in other areas of living. Flex your muscles and come on. You are really ready to break out of your fat cell now.

HOLISTIC LIFESTYLE CHANGE 3

You can be in the driver's seat with some Attitude Control. Here are some positive statements which will help you overcome your problem with sugar. Say them aloud and add any others you might think of:

1. My sugar preference was learned. I don't have to live for sugar and a sweet taste.
2. There is strong evidence that my sugar addiction has a significant effect on my mind and body. I'd rather be safe than wait for scientific proof.
3. I will not be afraid to change my food patterns.
4. It is important to act on new knowledge which will improve my whole body.
5. I belive that I can do anything I really want to do.
6. It is really worth trying.

Chapter Four

The Assertive You: ("When you laugh at me, I won't laugh back.")

"Hey, FAT STUFF!" That raucous voice calling to me in my high school hallway and the loud laughter of other students all around me still echo down the corridors of my memory more than thirty years later. I died a little each time that scene was replayed, and it was replayed many times. But what causes me even greater agony is that I also remember one of the loudest of those laughing voices was my own — me, being a good sport. No wonder I was voted "Most Generous" in my high school class. For four years I had handed over my self-esteem and participated in my own humiliation.

That wasn't the only time I allowed people to bully me because of my size. And I'm not the only overweight who has done so. As a group, one doctor told me, overweights are more easily manipulated than thins. Even after I lost 100 pounds, I was in the habit of acting passively. I had to learn a new kind of technique, called assertiveness, before I started sending out the message to others that I wouldn't be bullied. Unknowingly, for years I'd taught other people by my own behavior that they could treat me in an undignified way and I would take it. But I had to stand up and take the risk a behavior change always entails. At first my big question was, "Wouldn't people who were used to the old passive Jeane find the new me offensive?"

Dr. Wayne W. Dyer, who literally wrote the book on being effectively assertive, says in his *Pulling Your Own Strings:* "Many people assume that being assertive means being unpleasant, but it doesn't. It means making bold, confident declarations in defense of your rights. You can learn the art of disagreeing without being disagreeable, and you can stand up for yourself without being cantankerous."

There was my answer. Assertive behavior didn't mean becoming aggressive, it meant finding a livable halfway point between passive and aggressive. As for what others would think, Dr. Dyer had an answer for that quandary, too. "Whenever you find yourself

41

standing up for what you believe and wondering what everyone else is thinking," he says, "rest assured that if you took a private poll, you would find almost everyone secretly pulling for you, and admiring your attitude of toughness."

Becoming more assertive, if you are overweight, is just another way you can realize your creative potential and finally break out of your fat cell. Equally important, you will find you'll lose more weight if you treat yourself with dignity and expect better treatment from others.

Assertiveness: Why You Really Need It

Dr. Collie Conoley at the University of Texas recently made an interesting discovery when he studied the effects of assertive behavior on food intake. He found that giving assertiveness training to overweight women caused them to alter their food intake and lose weight. And this, in spite of the fact than most of the women didn't think assertiveness was very important. It doesn't seem to matter whether you value assertiveness or not. If you practice it, you will increase your self-esteem and lose weight.

Why are the overweight less aggressive as a group than thins? Psychologists have found that we generally avoid outward aggression because we've been taught (oh, so carefully) to "know our place." Even though we have strong egos we tend to be dominated by circumstances. We also have a low level of adaptation to new social situations; in other words, we don't know how to act. These conclusions point to a need for techniques which overweights can use to help them act assertively (in their own best interests) in a variety of daily activities, at home, on the job, in public and with themselves. In this chapter, you'll be able to determine just how assertive you are and what area of your life needs improvement. In Chapter Five, you will learn how to handle specific living problems with new assertiveness and dignity.

Remember, being nonassertive, like being overweight, is not your fault; it is a problem and problems have solutions. To develop your personal assertiveness program, the first step will be to determine your own Assertiveness Quotient.

Assertive Behavior Assessment*

The following statements will help you assess your A.Q. (Assertiveness Quotient) in four major areas of your life. If an item describes a situation unfamiliar to you, try to imagine your response. Check the number that best describes you and try to be as honest as you can. (Don't worry about the letters SI and LS after each question at this time. You will be using them later.)

* Developed in association with Dr. Trudy Helmlinger, Sacramento, California.

Inner Assertiveness

		Never	Rarely	Sometimes	Usually	Always	
1.	I do my own diet-thinking and make my own health decisions.	1	2	3	4	5	SI
2.	I can be myself around wealthy, prestigious or thin people.	1	2	3	4	5	SI
3.	I readily admit my mistakes and never blame them on my diet.	1	2	3	4	5	SI
4.	I accept responsibility for my life and my weight.	1	2	3	4	5	SI
5.	I make decisions and accept consequences.	1	2	3	4	5	SI
6.	When someone criticizes me constructively, I listen to the criticism without being defensive.	1	2	3	4	5	SI
7.	If I am jealous, I explore the reasons for my feelings and look for ways to increase my self-confidence and self-esteem.	1	2	3	4	5	SI
8.	When I am feeling insecure, I assess my personal strengths and then take positive action designed to make me feel more secure.	1	2	3	4	5	SI
9.	I generally express what I feel.	1	2	3	4	5	SI
10.	I do not interpret *every* comment as criticism.	1	2	3	4	5	SI

Inner Assertiveness Score Total

KEY: 10-20, You've been "had"; 20-35, you're better than you think you are; 35-45, assertive with a few slips; 45 and over, good inner assertiveness skills.

Family Assertiveness

		Never	Rarely	Sometimes	Usually	Always	
1.	I communicate my belief that everyone in the home should help with the upkeep rather than doing all myself in an impossible attempt to please.	1	2	3	4	5	LS

2. I make sexual advances toward my husband/
   wife or sex partner, because I believe I am
   truly desirable and lovable.   1 2 3 4 5   SI
3. When a spouse makes plans for me without
   my knowledge or consent, I am able to state
   why I cannot go along with them.   1 2 3 4 5   LS
4. I tell my children the things I like about them.   1 2 3 4 5   SI
5. When my family makes endless demands on
   my time and energy, I establish some firm
   notions about the amount of time I am willing
   to give.   1 2 3 4 5   LS
6. If my husband called to tell me he was bringing
   home an unexpected guest for dinner and I
   was very tired, I would level with him about my
   feelings and request that he make alternative
   plans.   1 2 3 4 5   LS
7. When my family (or friends) freely give diet
   advice, I express appreciation for their interest
   and concern without feeling obligated to
   follow their suggestions.   1 2 3 4 5   LS
8. I accept my spouse's interest in other people
   without feeling I must compete with them.   1 2 3 4 5   SI
9. I do not keep my mouth shut for the sake of
   "peace."   1 2 3 4 5   LS
10. I do not jump up and down to serve my family
    once I'm seated for a meal but insist that
    those wanting special service perform it for
    themselves.   1 2 3 4 5   LS

Family Assertiveness Score Total

KEY: 10-20, a "doormat"; 20-35, borderline assertive; 35-45, generally assertive; 45 and over, excellent family assertiveness skills.

Job Assertiveness

Never Rarely Sometimes Usually Always

1. My boss calls me by my first name; I call my
   boss by his/her first name.   1 2 3 4 5   LS
2. I have the self-confidence to quit a job that
   makes me miserable.   1 2 3 4 5   SI
3. I exude confidence at job interviews and insist
   on referring probing health (read weight)
   questions to my doctor.   1 2 3 4 5   SI

44

4. When I need help on the job, I can ask for it.   1 2 3 4 5   SI
5. When confused, I can ask for clarification because I do not accept the premise that overweights are dumb.   1 2 3 4 5   SI
6. I can ask for a promotion based on my performance.   1 2 3 4 5   SI
7. If I am underpaid, I ask for a salary increase without apology for my extra pounds.   1 2 3 4 5   SI
8. When working at a job or task I dislike intensely, I look for ways to improve my situation and never accept misery as just deserts for my overweight.   1 2 3 4 5   SI
9. When a subordinate completes a task for me with which I am dissatisfied, I ask that it be done again.   1 2 3 4 5   LS
10. If I hear that one of my co-workers is making remarks about my physical appearance, I would not hesitate to "have it out with him/her."   1 2 3 4 5   LS

Job Assertiveness Score Total ☐

KEY: 10-20, no promotion likely; 20-35, getting better but still not front office; 35-45, generally respected by co-workers; 45 and over, good job assertiveness skills.

Social Assertiveness

	Never	Rarely	Sometimes	Usually	Always	

1. I am poised and confident among slender strangers because I know my weight has nothing whatever to do with my worth.   1 2 3 4 5   SI
2. I freely express my emotions without fear that they will be dismissed because I am fat.   1 2 3 4 5   SI
3. I am friendly and considerate toward others, regardless of *their* size.   1 2 3 4 5   SI
4. I accept compliments without embarrassment or self-derision.   1 2 3 4 5   SI
5. I freely express my admiration of others' ideas and achievements.   1 2 3 4 5   SI
6. I never say "I'm sorry" when I have done nothing wrong.   1 2 3 4 5   SI
7. I take the initiative in personal contacts.   1 2 3 4 5   SI
8. I never apologize to others for my size.   1 2 3 4 5   SI

9. When I have done something well, I tell others. 1 2 3 4 5   SI

10. When at fault, I apologize for the fault — not for the fault *and* my weight. 1 2 3 4 5   SI

11. When I like someone very much, I tell them so without fear they will reject me because I am not perfect. 1 2 3 4 5   SI

12. When someone is annoying me with too many personal questions, I tell that person "It's none of your business." 1 2 3 4 5   LS

13. When someone cuts in front of me in line, I protest. 1 2 3 4 5   LS

14. When treated unfairly, or only as a "weight" and not a person, I object. 1 2 3 4 5   LS

15. I complain to the management when I have been overcharged, received poor service or been the butt of sarcastic comments. 1 2 3 4 5   LS

16. If something in my house or apartment malfunctions, I see that the landlord repairs it. 1 2 3 4 5   LS

17. If I am disturbed by someone smoking, drinking or eating my "binge" food in front of me, I say so. 1 2 3 4 5   LS

18. If a friend betrays my confidence, I tell that person how I feel. 1 2 3 4 5   LS

19. I ask my doctor all of the nutrition and health questions for which I want answers. 1 2 3 4 5   SI

20. I insist my doctor treat me as a thinking adult and not as a naughty child. 1 2 3 4 5   LS

21. I ask others for directions when I need help in finding my way. 1 2 3 4 5   SI

22. I do not cut off a relationship just because there are problems, but I never accept abuse about my size as the price for love or friendship. 1 2 3 4 5   SI

23. When at a restaurant I am served food that is not prepared the way I ordered it, I can express my dissatisfaction to the food server, regardless of my weight. 1 2 3 4 5   LS

24. Even though a clothes store clerk goes to a great deal of trouble finding my size for me, I am able to say "no" if I do not really want to purchase the merchandise. 1 2 3 4 5   LS

25. If I discover that I have purchased defective merchandise, I return it to the store. 1 2 3 4 5   LS

26. When people talk too loudly in a theater, lecture or concert, I am able to ask them to be quiet. 1 2 3 4 5   LS

27. I maintain good eye contact in conversations

because I have nothing of which to be
ashamed.

28. I would sit in front of a large group when the only
remaining seats are located there.   1 2 3 4 5   SI

29. I would speak to my neighbors when their dog is
keeping me awake with its barking.   1 2 3 4 5   LS

30. When I am interrupted while speaking, I
comment on the interruption and then finish
what I am saying.   1 2 3 4 5   LS

31. If I miss someone, I tell him/her that I want to
spend more time with that person.   1 2 3 4 5   SI

32. If a friend asks me to loan something and I really
don't want to, I turn down the request.   1 2 3 4 5   LS

33. If a friend invites me to join him/her and I really
don't want to, I turn down the request.   1 2 3 4 5   LS

34. When friends call and talk too long on the phone,
I can terminate the conversation effectively. 1 2 3 4 5 LS

35. When people are discussing overweight or diet
and I disagree with their points of view, I can express my difference of opinion.   1 2 3 4 5   LS

36. When someone makes demands on me that I
don't wish to fulfill, I resist the demands. 1 2 3 4 5   LS

37. I speak up readily in group situations.   1 2 3 4 5   SI

38. When one friend is not meeting all of my needs, I
establish meaningful ties with other people. 1 2 3 4 5   SI

39. I can express anger toward members of the opposite sex, as well as members of my own sex. 1 2 3 4 5 SI

40. I have a friend to whom I can tell virtually
anything.   1 2 3 4 5   SI

Social Assertiveness Score Total

KEY: 40-80, a real "patsy"; 80-140, better but needs to say "no" more often;
140-180, good social assertiveness most of the time; 180-200, assertiveness
genius.

Check your scores carefully. Now write what they mean in the
space provided below.

A.Q. Score   **Meaning**

Inner Assertiveness _____   _____

Family Assertiveness _____   _____

Job Assertiveness _____   _____

Social Assertivenes _____   _____

What do you see? Are you strong in one or more areas of assertiveness and weak in others? Perhaps you will be able to transfer the skills you have in one area to another, gradually becoming the assertive person you and others admire. Remember you were not born with a high A.Q., but you can become an absolute Einstein of assertiveness if you work at it.

Now go back once again to your answers on the Assertive Behavior Assessment. There are two hidden messages in those answers which can give you additional insights into how much self-iniative you have and how good you are at setting limits, two behaviors, you'll agree, that are valuable to any dieter.

Here's how you dig out this information. Add together all the answers labeled SI (Self-initiative) and put the total on the correct line below. Do the same for the answers labeled LS (Limit-setting).

Score   **Meaning**

Self-initiative _____   _____

Limit Setting _____   _____

KEY: (SI) Self-initiative, 40-80, "can't get off the dime"; 80-120, some initiative, but not ready to climb Mt. Everest; 120-160, a self-starter most of the time; 160-200, Mr./Ms. Success!

KEY: (LS) Limit-setting, 30-60, "People walk all over me"; 60-90, spend too much energy "people-pleasing"; 90-120, show a moderate-to-good ability to set limits; 120-150, you let people know just how you want to be treated.

Of course, the higher you scored on self-initiative and limit setting, the more assertive you are. But there is a Catch-22 in scoring high in the self-initiative area. Generally speaking, people who score 160-180 tend toward compulsiveness. They try to prove their worth, but never quite make it, at least in their own eyes. They tend not to feel comfortable no matter what heights they scale. Nevertheless, it may be an acceptable trade-off, since these success-oriented people high in assertiveness and self-initiative also firmly believe they can accomplish what they set out to do. They have an enhanced ability to risk goal-setting; they go after what they secretly want.

On the other hand, the meaning of your score in the area of limit-setting is quite straight forward. The lower you score the more likely you are to be the person everybody kicks around; the higher you score the more you really believe your rights are as valid as the next person's.

What does all this mean to the overweight? Simply this. It seems reasonable to assume that assertive, self-initiating people and limit-setting people are also people who have a better chance at grabbing the brass ring of life, and that means losing weight and keeping it off.

Assertiveness Workshops for the Overweight

These tests were administered to several groups of overweight women along with a basic lecture on assertiveness. Most of the women, who belong to Overeaters Anonymous groups, agreed that they were far more assertive than they had been a few years earlier before participating in OA's group sessions. Over 90 percent of the women admitted that merely taking the test had made them more aware of some harmful passive behavior which they wanted to begin to change. The highest A.Q. scores were made in the job area, since many of the women were high achievers in business. The lowest scores were made in the social area, where ability seems to count for less than physical appearance. One women remarked that being able to answer *always* to Number 14 on the Social Assertiveness test ("When treated unfairly, or only as a 'weight' and not a person, I object.") was as assertive as any fat person could possibly get. "If you can answer *always* to that one," she said, "you don't even have to take the rest of the test. From now on that is the standard of assertiveness I want to set for myself."

The ABC's of Assertiveness

If you have determined that you are not going to let anybody, let alone everybody, walk all over you, what's your next move — become a black belt in karate? Of course not. Don't make the mistake of thinking assertive means aggressive. Actually they are two very different kinds of behavior and you should be particularly careful not to confuse the two. According to Dr. Peter Lindner of the Lindner Clinic in Los Angeles, confusing aggression for assertiveness is the biggest problem the overweight have with assertiveness training. "When the overweight become aggressive," says the doctor, "it backfires on them, and their self-esteem suffers a setback."

The fact is that aggressive behavior doesn't work; it only increases the opportunities others have to be abusive toward you and that will make you feel bad about yourself. Assertive behavior, on the other hand, puts you in control of a situation. You can choose to go as far as you want or not go very far at all. Again you are up in the driver's seat, just where you belong, just where you've always wanted to be. First, you will need to know just what behavioral responses you have been using.

There are three ways you can act when you are dealing with other people: passively, aggressively or assertively. Most fat people, psychologists say, are passive. When someone treats us unfairly, calls us names or otherwise tramples on our human rights, we tend to:

1. Say nothing.
2. Abuse ourselves to show what good sports we are.
3. Get our feelings hurt.
4. Be angry, but swallow the angry feelings (along with a lot of unnecessary food).
5. Give the person a dirty look.

Next there is aggressive behavior. Sometimes when we overweights lose our weight or just get tired of taking abuse about it, our first reaction is to want to get even. Here's what we might do:

1. We go on the attack with YOU messages. "Well, you aren't so good-looking yourself. Look at that bald head/paunch/low-paying job/bratty children/bad marriage, etc.!"
2. We express other negative opinions about the other person's looks, intelligence, sexiness, ability or ancestry.
3. We overreact and try for the big "put down."
4. We confront in a bitter, angry way, which is likely to leave us feeling guilty. And feeling guilty is even more likely to lead to an overeating binge.

Finally there is assertive behavior. This is the ideal lifestyle goal of overweights, indeed of any person who wants to be able to experience relationships with honest self-expression. Here is how you can deal assertively with one instance of verbal hostility with which we're all familiar.

Hostile statement: "My, you're fat. How much *do* you weigh, anyway?

Response: State your feelings, firmly telling the other person how you want them to act in the future. Example: "I do not feel good when you discuss my weight, and I don't want you to do it again."

What if the abuser ignores you? Here is an assertive escalation technique to overcome continued verbal aggression.

1. Low level assertiveness — Make a polite statement of limits or request the person to stop intruding. Examples: "I do not discuss my weight," or "I do not like to answer personal questions, please do not ask again."

2. Intensify — If verbal aggressiveness continues, repeat your request increasing verbal intensity. Example: "I never discuss my weight, and I do not want you to discuss it."

3. Consequence — If abuse continues, inform the person that further intrusion will result in a consequence. Example: "I do not discuss my weight and I do not want you to discuss it. If you insist on this, I will leave."

4. Carry out the consequence — If the clod still doesn't get your message, *leave.*

In Chapter Five, we will discuss the assertive escalation and other techniques in depth, using a number of verbal situations overweights commonly experience in their relationships with other people. You may never have to use most of them, but you will be ready with a tool that really works should the necessity arise.

What If People Don't Like the Assertive You?

One of the most frequent questions asked by workshop participants (including myself) was: what if my family, friends or boss get angry at me for asserting myself?

Rationalizing that we might lose the affection of those we care about is one of the ways we overweights talk ourselves out of assertive behavior. It is true that there will be times when you won't get a positive response. People who have been used to manipulating you for their own purposes may have temper tantrums or quit speaking to you. You could lose a job (chance are, if your job depended on your boss's browbeating you, it wasn't a good job to begin with), or even a mate. These extremes of reacting to your becoming a wholly integrated, self-respectful and dignified person are rare and usually mean the relationship was a destructive one for you in the first place. Most people will rapidly adjust to the new assertive you, and your most intimate relationships will improve as long as you maintain a good level of assertiveness. What happens if you assert yourself for a time, then fall back on the old patterns of behavior? All your relationships will revert to the old passive/aggressive patterns. If you want the benefits, you have to keep it up until assertiveness becomes second nature.

You're Going to Feel Good About Yourself

The more assertive and less passive and aggressive you become, the more you will be lacking in your own best interests. The assertive person, as Dr. Lindner points out, is completely in charge. You will feel capable and confident in the face of hostility or cockiness. You will value your own opinion and be able to express it without fear. You will be able to take full responsibility for your behavior. You will give to yourself the right to be yourself, without guilt. Your assertiveness will greatly enhance your own self-esteem. After you have behaved in an assertive manner you will be able to say, "I respect myself for that."

Be assured that assertiveness will not turn you into a "pushy" selfish person; it will turn you into a person you and others admire. Think of the people you admire. Does anyone walk all over them?

At this point, you probably have a question. How, you ask, can a fat person with a low estimation of self-worth change his or her passive behavior and begin to act assertively? Perhaps you believe you ought to wait until you have a better self-image. The answer is so simple most of us don't even think of it: *BEHAVE ASSERTIVELY FIRST* and you will get rid of your poor self-image; get rid of your poor self-image and you will be able to shed weight.

Action is the magic word.

When you strive to become assertive you are merely setting standards of behavior for yourself. Some interesting research has been done regarding the overweight and standard-setting. Psychologists at Emory University in Atlanta, Georgia divided dieting overweight subjects into several groups. One group set standards of behavior for themselves. Two other groups didn't. You can guess what happened. According to a research extract, the standard-setting group experienced "significantly greater weight loss," which resulted in increased awareness of their behavior toward food and the ability to self-correct when they made mistakes. Of nineteen different techniques offered the three groups, standard-setting was rated highest by the participants themselves.

Set standards of assertive behavior for yourself today. Say "I will go this far and no farther." You might want to use the Bill of

Rights on page 54, developed by members of my assertiveness workshop for the overweight as a place to start. Start where you can, but start.

You are now well on the road to healing your mind and body of the ills of self-blame, self-humiliation and the erroneous belief that you are always wrong because you are still overweight. Believing that extra pounds somehow made you less a human being with less than a human being's rights on this earth literally made your whole body sick. Acting and believing deeply that you are worthwhile, that your life has meaning and that there is hope for the future will make you whole and well again.

You have to love yourself. It will make all the difference. You are not trapped by the circumstances of life. You have the ability to become untrapped whenever you say so. Sure you have made mistakes, but you are trying to deal with them and grow from them. Best of all, you have something important that you don't even know you have. You have the ability to take charge of your life as soon as you give yourself permission to do so.

Now that you are beginning to assert your rights as a person, no matter what your size, you are beginning to live a little more sanely and meaningfully because you are taking the responsibility for your own behavior. As you practice asserting your feelings, you will learn how to handle your weight problem better than you ever have before. Never again will you take abuse, then go home and eat over it. You are coming closer to the day when you will clang the door shut on your lonely fat cell forever.

In this chapter you have formed an idea of what assertiveness is all about and learned from your A.Q. test the areas in your life you need to work on. In the next chapter, you will read about some real-life assertive techniques which have worked for other overweights in their daily relationships. Best of all, you will discover, as I did, that when others laugh at you, the last thing in the world you have to do is laugh at yourself.

An Overweight Person's Assertive Bill of Rights

1. I have the right to be thin.
2. I have the right to health privacy.
3. I have the right to set my own natural weight.
4. I have the right to reject food I don't want.
5. I have the right to compete for any job for which I qualify.
6. I have the right to reply to rudeness.
7. I have the right to be who I am whatever my size.
8. I have the right to put myself first.
9. I have the right to be ambitious for myself.
10. I have rights and the right to stand up for them.

HOLISTIC LIFESTYLE CHANGE 4

Today:

1. I will treat myself with respect, saying not one derogatory word about my size.

2. I will reject the "Most Generous" award if it is paid for with my dignity.

3. I will remember that my A.Q. score can be changed and use the quiz as a starting point toward assertive personhood.

4. I will make a list of four people I admire and decide whether they are passive, aggressive or assertive.

Chapter Five

Winning the Respect You Deserve

"If you want to change what other
people think of you, you must change
what you think of yourself."
— George Bernard Shaw

To have the kind of self-esteem Shaw was talking about requires you to set a high value on yourself which you will allow no one to undermine. Before you can learn assertive ways of dealing with the everyday problems that cause you loss of self-esteem, you must learn to see thin chauvinistic put-downs for what they really are — verbal cruelties for which you should feel contempt, not self-blame. It is not always easy to recognize thin chauvinists; they come in many disguises. But you must be able to see through their masks if you intend to succeed with your holistic, mind-body plan to lose weight permanently. Be on the lookout for and on your guard against these types:

The Joker: The function of the joker is to make you the butt of fat stereotype jokes and then expect you to laugh with him. "Heard the one about the fat lady in the telephone booth?" he asks. "No offense," he goes on, nudging you with his elbow. "Only a joke." You are not expected to be angry, but to acquiesce like a good sport. Good Sportism is expected of the overweight. It's as American as apple, pardon the analogy, pie. The thin chauvinistic joker is not a new phenomenon. Back in 1863, a fat man ran for governor of Ohio, providing the electorate with a couple of belly laughs. His opponents circulated this jingle about his size: "If flesh is grass, as people say, then Johnny Brough's a load of hay." On hearing this, John Brough retorted, "Guess I am hay, the way asses keep nibbling at me." He was elected.

The Helper: This thin chauvinist's cruelty comes wrapped in a righteous disguise. "I'm only telling you this for your own good," she says, after commenting with surprise about your weight. The Helpers would never dream of making a similar comment about another kind of physical problem. You never hear them say, "Gee, your goiter has grown again!" or "Your limp is much worse than it was, isn't it?" or "My, your bosom is as flat as ever!"

The Name Caller: Even in this day of relaxed etiquette, it is still gross to call a person by any name other than his or her own. The uncouth individual who insists on yelling, "Hey, Chubby," "Fatty," or "Tank," should be confronted. Insist that you will only respond to your proper name, *and stick to it.*

The Tempter: This form of thin chauvinism parades as kindness such as, "Go ahead, have a piece of cake. I won't tell a soul." The issue, of course, is not a piece of cake, but the inability of the thin chauvinist to treat an overweight's wishes seriously.

The Patronizer: It sounds like honest praise but it is really a superior put-down. "That's a good, dark color for you, my dear. It's so slenderizing."

The Gossip: This thin chauvinist comes bearing cruel words disguised as news. "You know your wife is so worried about your weight, she doesn't know what to do."

The Business Bigot: Personnel managers, especially, think this is letting you down easy. They usually say something like, "You'd be so much happier out of the front office and in the stockroom."

The Sarcastic: "Want to lose ten ugly pounds? Cut off your head!" Cruelty masquerading as irony often is only thinly-veiled hostility.

The Cat: The thin chauvinist Cat is really out to undercut the attention you're being paid. "So you've lost thirty pounds. Was that *all* you had to lose?"

There is never an excuse for criticizing someone for excess pounds. It is not only tactless but illogical since such lack of respect for an individual's health problem is more apt to hinder than help. The important thing for you to remember is: YOU DON'T HAVE TO TAKE IT ANYMORE! You have the right to health privacy.

Preparing For the New Assertive You

There are a few steps you can take to prepare yourself to exercise assertiveness in your life.

1. Make sure you don't lack a basic self-respect so that you will not be *inviting* disrespect from others. Never put yourself down in front of others (or even in your own mind) or you will be as much as issuing a call to any bully within hearing distance. Why not enhance your growing self-respect with the new and more positive vocabulary you'll find on page 68.

2. Pat yourself on the back for the good things about you. Appreciate yourself. In this way you will be reinforcing your own best behavior in your own mind. Let's face it, a lot of damage is done to the best weight-losing program right in our own minds.

3. Dress yourself with pride. Wearing any old thing just because you're overweight and think you don't deserve anything better is just about the least respectful thing you can do to yourself.

4. Come out of the closet and dare to do some of the things you have always wanted to do. Sure it is safer to hide, for the moment anyway, but lack of social interaction will catch up with you some day. If you want to do something, do it today.

5. Learn to forgive yourself, as Dr. Sheldon Kopp says, "again, and again and again." Don't constantly remind yourself of all the mistakes you have made in the past. Try to learn the words, "I forgive me," and make them a part of your everyday life.

6. Get a feel of who you are as a human being. Get in touch with the *self* that is you. "This being of mine," said Marcus Aurelius, "consists of a little flesh, a little breath and *the part that governs.*"

You are about to learn techniques that will help you govern, help you take charge, of your own life. In the final analysis, aren't you living with yourself? You are going to be much more comfortable with the assertive you.

An Assertive, Dignified Defense

When you have become the target of negative energy in the form of put-downs about your size, remember that you have a right to be you and not allow yourself to be manipulated. Here are some situations with which overweights often have to deal, along with a sample assertive response, so that you can maintain your diet and your self-esteem.

Family Holidays

Mother It's so nice to have you home again, dear. I've made your favorite banana cake.

You: I'm sorry, Mother, I'm not eating sugar calories.

Mother: But I made it *just for you!*

You: I realize you went to a lot of trouble, but I am no longer eating sweet foods.

Mother: Surely, one little bite won't hurt.

You: You may be right, Mother, but I am no longer eating sugar and I don't want you to make any more desserts for me. I'll have a fine dinner with all the other good things you've cooked. You do want me to look and feel better, don't you?

Mother: How can you ask such a thing? Of course, I do.

You: Thank you, Mother. I knew I could count on your help.

This conversation may seem a bit simplistic and probably somewhat shorter than the real thing, but it makes the point that if you remain in control and refuse tó be manipulated, you will have nothing to regret after your next home-baked holiday.

Take another look at the family portion of the Assertiveness Quiz in Chapter Four. Can you see any situation in which this technique would have given you a higher score?

In the Office

He: Here, have a chair. Have *two* chairs. Ha! Ha! That's a joke, pal.

You: I don't think that is funny. I only want one chair.

He: You don't have to get upset about it. It was just harmless fun.

You: I can see how you'd think that, but I still don't believe it's funny. I only want one chair.

He: You're not being a very good sport. Can't you take a joke?

You: Yes, I like a good joke, but I don't think jokes about my size are funny. I only want one chair.

He: I can't talk to you. You sound like a broken record.

You: Yes, that must be how I sound, but I still want only one chair.

One of the most important aspects of being verbally assertive is to persist in stating how you feel and what you want, without getting angry.

Go back to the job section of the Assertiveness Quiz in the last chapter. Could you use this technique to improve your overall score?

At a Restaurant

Waiter: Good evening. We have a very good lasagna special tonight.

You: I would like the baked fish, please, with a green cooked vegetable instead of the potato, and no dressing on my salad.

Waiter: (With an obvious shrug) I can bring you rice instead of the potato.

You: No, I prefer a nonstarchy vegetable. Do you have green beans or asparagus?

Waiter: I don't know. It's not on the menu.

You: Please check with the chef.

Later

Waiter: (Looking harassed) The chef has substituted cottage cheese for the potato.

You: That will not do. I want a cooked vegetable and please exchange this salad for one *without* dressing.

Waiter: (Angry) I'll try.

Later

Waiter: Here is your order — baked fish, green beans and a salad with no dressing.

You: Thank you. I like a restaurant that is flexible enough to give me what I want.

Waiter: Enjoy your dinner, Madam.

The customer is *always* right. You have a perfect right to have food prepared as you order it. If it is not done to your satisfaction, you have the right to return it until it conforms with your needs. After all, you are buying. Don't get side-tracked trying to please the waiter or any other person who is offering you a service for which you pay. You are the one to be pleased.

How did you answer question 23 in the Social Assertiveness portion of the Assertive Behavior Assessment Quiz in Chapter Four? If you score one, two or three, this technique might be worth a try next time you find yourself in a restaurant.

Shopping for Clothes

You: I would like to see something in a straight skirt.

Salesclerk: Honey, you can't wear a straight skirt. Let me show you something in an A-line from the Matron Shop.

You: No, I do not like the A-line style. I want to see a straight skirt in my size, please.

Salesclerk: All right, but I don't think it's any use. *You* people need an A-line.

You: I want to see the store manager.

Salesclerk: You don't have to get huffy, and make trouble for me.

Manager: May I help you?

You: I expect you can. I came into the store to buy a straight skirt. Your clerk insists on showing me an A-line and used a derogatory manner toward me. I must be treated politely or I will not shop here.

Manager: You are absolutely right. Our policy is always to treat our customers with courtesy. I'm sure this is all an unfortunate misunderstanding.

Salesclerk: Yes sir, I did not understand. I have a lovely straight skirt in her size, and I'll be happy to show it to her.

You: Thank you. Please bring it to the fitting room.

Salesclerk: Right away, Ma'am.

It is your right to *make up your own mind* about what you will or will not wear. It is also your right by your behavior to *demand* courteous treatment. You do not have to take sarcasm from prejudiced nitwits.

How did you score on Statement 15 in the social assertiveness part of the quiz in the last chapter? How would you score now?

At a Group Meeting:

Member: I still can't believe you lost so much weight. It was over a hundred pounds, wasn't it?

You: Yes. Have you read the new Irwin Shaw novel? I thought it was his best yet, and I've been recommending it to all my friends.

Member: Oh, how I wish I could lose ten pounds before Christmas. I think I'll come over and sit by you so that some of your magic will rub off on me.

You: There's no magic to it. Overweight was a health problem which I worked on with my doctor, my diet group and myself. Now, I'm trying to build a new life with new interests. Have you seen the symphony's new conductor in action? He is a fine interpreter of the Baroque masters.

Later

Members: (In chorus) Look at her! She's turning down dessert again. What willpower! I wish I had some. I'm barely squeezing into my size 5's.

You: I appreciate all the support you have given my weight loss and I understand that your comments are meant to praise me. But I want to get on with my new life without always having to discuss dieting. I would rather talk about the group business. Why don't we plan a crafts fair to raise money for our scholarship fund?

There are times when you want to be assertive but in a low-key manner. This form of thin chauvinism is really well-intentioned, if misplaced, and requires from you some persistent, but gentle, re-education. If you continue to insist on a change of topic, the group will gradually accommodate you. Unfortunately, they will probably admire your strong character, too, ("Oh, she lost so much weight, but she never wants to talk about it.") and you'll be elected president the next term.

At Home

You: I've found a new way of eating that I really want to do.

Family: Another diet! That means we're all going to starve.

You: No, I will be cooking more healthful meals, because that is the way I want to eat.

Family: You'll never fix desserts, and the holidays are coming. Can't you wait and start the first of the year?

You: No, it's important to me that I start today.

Family: Why do we have to suffer, just because you eat too much?

You: I can see how you'd think my weight is my fault, but I am going to begin eating differently today.

Family: We want you to be thinner. Why can't you just cut down on your own sweets, but keep baking for us?

You: I feel it's too much temptation to have those foods in the house. Why don't you have your dessert during lunch at school and at work? I am going to start a new way of eating today, and I won't be baking sugary things.

Family: That's sure selfish of you. Other mothers and wives wouldn't do that. They put their families first.

You: It may look selfish to you, but this new way of eating for a healthy mind and body is what I'm starting today.

Family: Well, O.K., but we don't understand.

You: It is a mystery why some people get fat and others don't, but I'm taking charge of my health today in a new holistic way.

Family: Is that some new kind of diet?

You: In a way. We can learn about the holistic health movement together, as I begin to eat differently for my mind and body.

Family: Oh, O.K., but it sure sounds complicated.

You: It isn't. It's the most natural way of living, and, best of all, I'm starting it today.

Check the Family Assertiveness Quiz in Chapter Four. Are you being manipulated by your family?

The manipulators (and families are masters) have learned all the right guilt buttons to push. They have always worked before, but this time they won't work. You have the right to make up your own mind about your life. You don't need to apologize for health decisions you make about your body; you don't need to argue or justify your new lifestyle. Remember, you have the right to put yourself first at times, and this is one of those times.

When you think back, you can remember many instances when

you were badly treated because you *allowed* it to happen out of a sense of guilt for being fat in the first place. One woman in an assertiveness workshop told her brother-in-law how much she weighed each time he asked (usually in a public place), because she thought if she weighed that much, she *had* to admit it. You can see how difficult assertive behavior would be, if you hung on to guilt. *You are not to blame for becoming overweight, you are only responsible for taking charge of your health today.* Try to etch that message into your brain so that guilt and self-blame (false, in any case) cannot be manipulated by others.

A caution: Although it happens rarely, there are times in everyone's life when even the best methods don't work. A very few people are such clods that all the saints working together couldn't get through their ironclad sensibility. In situations in which a person does not respond to your assertive attempts or becomes threatening, I certainly believe in self-defense as opposed to fat martyrdom. "I don't advocate psychoanalyzing a person as I'm falling to the floor," says psychologist Dr. Salvatore Didato. "If I must, as a last resort, I will respond in kind, but without going beyond the level of hostility that was presented to me."

On the other hand, you may not always have to use assertive techniques to get the good treatment you deserve. Sometimes all you have to do is look the other person straight in the eye, asking: "Don't you care that you're hurting my feelings?" That person may love you and care for you very deeply. Perhaps he or she has just formed a bad habit of talking about your weight and had no idea you cared so much. Very often such directness is all that is needed to change a bad habit into respectful behavior. Use your good judgment as to whether or not you need to use your new assertiveness in every situation.

What About Your Right to Public Assertiveness?

After you have practiced assertive techniques in your private life for a short time, you may begin to notice and resent fat prejudice in the public sector. For example, a well-known actress makes a derogatory remark about fat people on television, a colledge expels its overweight students, a classified ad specifies only thin, attractive candidates need apply or a researcher claims fat people are using up too much of the world's energy through overeating. You have a right to complain when public *big-otry* reflects on you. All of these prejudicial things happened and overweight people did assert themselves, writing letters, asking for apologies and boycotting products. *You don't have to take it anymore, anywhere!*

Coping with Compliments

Throughout most of this chapter you have been learning assertive ways to handle put-downs no matter where they come from. But how do you handle compliments? There comes a time in every overweight person's life when she or he has to be able to accept a compliment graciously and assertively. Many of us, used to negative treatment by thin chauvinists, have never learned how to handle a sincere compliment. Here are just two negative emotions about positive comments which can trigger problem eating instead of self-esteem.

As I said in *The Thin Book*, many overweights take compliments as guarded insults. We tend to look for the *hidden* negative meaning. Because we don't think well of ourselves, we can't believe that others sincerely find things praiseworthy about us.

Our other reaction to compliments is to disallow them completely. We think the complimenting party must be mistaken, and we immediately point out their mistake to them. For example:

Complimentor: That's a lovely dress you're wearing today.
You: What! This old thing. It's been hanging in my closet for years and actually is rather worn and faded.

There are dozens of other ways we put ourselves down, but you get the idea. Over the years we program ourselves to reject honest admiration. "I can't do anything right," we repeat to ourselves over and over until we believe it and, by our behavior, insist that everyone else believe it, too.

What nonsense! You do many things well. Chances are you are a high achiever in many areas of your life. Your problem is one of recognition. Why don't you try some self-recognition?

1. Select one of your many good points and compliment yourself on how well you perform. Tomorrow select another point, and the next day another.

2. Try not to be such a perfectionist. People who have a low sense of self-esteem are generally too hard on themselves. Reward yourself if you even come close to your high standards.

You can see that the reason a compliment embarrasses you into an immediate denial is that you have a conviction that there is nothing about you deserving a compliment. That is absolutely false. You merit compliments just like anyone else. You don't have to deny your good points because of your size. Begin as soon as you can to practice accepting compliments graciously by simply saying, "Thank you." For you, this will probably be extremely assertive behavior. Next, try an uncomplicated statement of gratitude, such as: "How nice of you to say so." Just that. Nothing more. Don't get elaborate, because at first you're going to be unaccustomed to it.

You will find it is all quite comfortable after a time and leaves you feeling good about yourself. You are behaving with poise and tact and you know it.

Asserting yourself, to yourself, as a person worthy of compliments is the other side of the coin to asserting yourself to others by demanding respectful treatment. You need both. You deserve both, so that you can break out of your lonely fat cell.

Avoiding the Good Sport Syndrome

One final word on Good Sportism, a system of behavior response so ingrained in the overweight it amounts to national brainwashing. You must never allow yourself to be convinced that your "Popularity" is worth your self-respect. That is too high a price to pay for momentary acceptance. And as you have learned by now, no one really likes a doormat.

The Good Sport Syndrome — being a "jolly fat victim" — was first defined by Marvin Grosswirth in his book *Fat Pride* when he called getting rid of Good Sportism a major step in building self-esteem. "You have to make a decision," Grosswirth said firmly, "that you will stop being a good sport even though our contemporary cultural media have been fostering the good sport as a national symbol and the bad sport as unpatriotic. What utter nonsense!"

Grosswirth goes further and urges overweights to abstain from participating in the prejudice parade whether it is Polish jokes, bald-headed cracks or midget stories. That shouldn't be too hard for us; after all we've been there.

How Assertiveness Fits Your Holistic Weight-losing Plan

I once asked a much-overweight member of a diet group what one word was the most important word in her life, naturally expecting to hear the word "thin," or at least the word "diet." Without hesitation she said, *"Peace."*

We fat people have lived for so long in conflict, conflict with others and conflict with our inner selves, that we literally crave peace as if it were the sweetest confection in the world. It is the one element that brings the joy of balance to our minds and bodies. Peace unifies. Peace is nonlimiting.

The assertive dieter is on the road to peace. "Aggression tramples," says Lois Lindauer of Diet Workshop fame, "assertion joins forces. Aggression creates hostility; assertion smooths the way. Aggression irritates, assertion soothes. Aggressors may be victors but asserters are *winners*."

It seems clear from even a cursory glance at the majority of weight-losing philosophies that creating a successful weight loss pattern means developing new social behavior. We overweights can no longer make it in today's world by either passive or "life-of-the-party" defenses. Both of these desperate ego-bolsterers have to be replaced with a permanent, positive self-image. For most of us this means learning how to say "yes," or "no," instead of just "me,too."

It seems as if one of the most important tools you can use in weight losing — right up there with a healthful eating plan — is assertiveness. It will give you the freedom to be who you really are, reducing external and internal pressures that urge you to conform to someone else's idea of you.

The most sought after medicine in the Middle Ages was ground Egyptian mummy or dried goat gallstones called bezoar. With these exotic potions, our ancestors believed that they could gain power over fear, evil spirits and other people. Today we need a potent, new medicine for our old yearning for self-mastery, and that medicine is assertiveness.

Monitor your body and mind as you begin to use assertive methods in your everyday life, and you will soon notice that you are getting positive signals after acting assertively. Your whole being feels better, physically and mentally. This self-awareness and heightened self-esteem, in turn, becomes an energy force which you can use to take charge of your life. When you are in charge, and you know it, you can decide to make changes. No one else can make these changes for you — there is no white knight in shining armor for any fat man or woman. You must develop the lifestyle that allows you to lose weight. Then go seek every method and resource you sense can help you.

The biggest bonus you will get from assertiveness is this: you will finally own your own behavior. No one else will be able to make you do anything you don't want to do. Whenever you don't like the behavior you have, you can change!

Don't think that assertiveness is ever beyond your abilities. Remember the lesson of the *Wizard of Oz*? The Scarecrow searched for a brain, the Tin Man for a heart and the Lion for courage, only to discover in the end that these qualities were part of them, *in* them, all the time. You will find when you risk being assertive that it was a talent you had all along; you just didn't know how to use it.

Now you have skills, and through additional reading (see the recommended reading list in this chapter) you can learn more techniques for applying assertive principles. You will be able to confront difficult situations without dreading them before, or eating over them afterwards. You are truly giving yourself priority, perhaps for the first time in your life, and gaining the respect from yourself and others you have always deserved. You are practicing the integrated, healing concept of holism.

In the next chapter, you will learn that it is possible to achieve a good body image from right where you are, so that you can remove one of the stumbling blocks on the road to happy wholeness.

Positive Vocabulary Primer

In order for you to be a successful dieter (or anything else), you must think well of yourself. All your life you have heard negative expressions about overweight, and you have used them against yourself. Now is the time to throw out these old negatives and begin to use positive expressions so you can begin to think of yourself in a new and more self-respectful way.

Fat Cell Words	Break Free Words
Big, fat slob	Junoesque, Samson-like
glutton, gluttonous	appetite, gusto, gourmand
socially immature	sensitive
jolly	joyous, exuberant, zesty, witty
sexless	sensual, flashy, abundant, curvy, voluptuous, superman, buxom, stacked, well-endowed
lazy	deliberate, prudent, energy-conservationist
dumb	cautious, thorough
too-sensitive	deep-feeling, expressive
bad	made a mistake, impulsive, misconstrued, went astray, stumbled, misjudged
weak	needs support

Your Assertiveness Reading List

Baer, Jean, *How to be an assertive (not aggressive) woman*, Signet, New York, 1976.
Lindner, Peter G., M.D., *It's Your Right to be Thin!* The Lindner Clinic, Box 2097, South Gate, California, 90280, 1977.
Smith, Manuel J., Ph.D., *When I say no, I feel guilty*, Bantam Books, New York, 1975.

Remember, when you begin to take charge of your life, you are going to be undertaking a new way of responding to life's pressures. You should watch out for old behavior habits which come sneaking back when you need them least, old habits which have taught others you can be, indeed want to be, manipulated.

1. *Stop asking others to take charge for you.*

   Your speech pattterns, including your vocabulary will be your biggest problem. Don't say, "Won't you please go to the mountains with me?" Say instead, "Let's go to the mountains."

2. *Do not surrender sole responsibility for your money.*

   Like it or not money equals power. When you allow someone to have power over your money, you are announcing that you want to be powerless.

3. *Learn to recognize your unhappy passive traits.*

   If you have been giving in just because you think it is expected, you are going to be uncomfortable, angry and, eventually, fatter.

4. *Take responsibility for mistakes.*

   Accept responsibility, then take steps to rectify your problem. In this way, you will never be able to rationalize that someone "forced" you to eat a dessert you didn't want to eat.

5. *Take risks when dealing with victimizers.*

   Asserting yourself is a risk, since you have taught others they could have their way with you for so long. Taking back your own life and making your own rules is less an ordeal than living a life others have chosen for you.

6. *Stop putting yourself down.*

   Never say, "I'm so dumb," or "I'm just a big, fat slob," or "I'm not very graceful." These put-downs are like handing out legal licenses for others to abuse you.

7. *Don't feel guilty for becoming assertive.*

   Too many people take back their assertiveness when others make them feel guilty. Watch out for those who say: "How could you do this after all I've done for you?" STAY IN CONTROL.

Chapter Six

Achieving a Positive Body Image

It's no news to you that the thin body is the ideal image to have in today's world. You face that fact every day at work, in your social life, and, most of all, in your mirror. The well-covered body (as my grandmother used to call it) is not admired as it once was, and not too long ago at that.

You need only go back to the turn of the twentieth century to find a voluptuous Lillian Russell the toast of New York. A little further back in time the beauties of Rubens and the other Renaissance painters had curves that undulated across huge canvasses. And if you go back far enough, but not quite to the Earth Mother, you will find that Cleopatra barged down the Nile, with Antony panting after her, wearing a body that would send her straight to a Jack LaLanne disaster unit today.

The full form, male or female, has historically been an object of envy because most people didn't have enough to eat. Today almost everyone in the Western world has enough to eat, so the opposite is admired — self-control and thinness to the point of emaciation. What this means to you is simply this: "in" body styles are a matter of fashion. To base your feelings of self-worth and self-love on the whims of taste is ridiculous.

You want very much to lose weight for your health and in order to feel comfortable in the age in which we live. Not many of us are so revolutionary we would choose to remain fat in a world made for the thin body. The point is that overweights who have a disturbed body image, one of which they are ashamed and disgusted, carry an almost insurmountable burden. It is next to impossible to integrate your mind and body in a holistic healing diet while you are consumed with physical self-loathing. You have to start living, wholly living, from where you are right now in order to have a chance at the thinner body you deserve.

There are many bars forged by the prison of your fat cell. One of them is called negative body image. You are about to break that one.

What Science Knows About Body Image

Surprise! The most serious body image distortion occurs among the very thin in *anorexia nervosa*, a psychological disorder where young women attempt to starve themselves because they think they are too fat. Next in line are overweight women who tend to see themselves as heavier than they really are and lastly, overweight men who perceive themselves as appearing lighter than they actually are.

The famous weight expert Dr. Alfred Stunkard and his associate Dr. M. Mendelson put together one of the most thorough body image studies of the obese. They discovered that only a minority of the adult-onset obese had body image disturbance. But for female subjects who were fat in adolescence, their poor body image persisted up to twenty years after they lost weight. Considering that the teen years are emotionally difficult in the first place, it is obvious that overweight at that stage of life amounts to a double whammy! If you were fat during adolescence, you will have work to do to adjust your body image to reality.

Negative body image is not just the problem of the too thin or too fat. In a *Psychology Today* survey of 62,000 readers (a highly educated and economically well-off readership), 55 percent of the women and 45 percent of the men had negative body images. One respondent from this highly sophisticated sampling put it this way: "I am 30 years old, a success in a field few women enter, happily married and valued by my family, but I'd chuck it all to be the kind of long-legged tawny beauty praised in myth and toothpaste ads." And you wonder that you have body image problems!

When it comes down to it, science knows two things for sure about improving body image for the overweight:

1. Body image automatically improves with maturity, according to a Fordham University study.

2. With weight loss, body image changes markedly for the better, but it can take years to adjust the mental body image to the reality of having a thin body.

You and Your Body

There is a strange dichotomy that rules the overweight in relation to their bodies; they are at once preoccupied with them, yet out of touch. While being consciously involved with dieting away pounds, we can, at the same time, float through life ignoring our bodies. We tend to say: "This body isn't really me. I am better than

70

this too-abundant flesh." A holistic approach to mind-body dieting means we will have to learn to connect our bodies with our inner self.

It is imperative, then, that we be thoroughly realistic about who we are physically. We have to learn to go well beyond the negative fat body image. In order to form a basis for liking our bodies, we must break down our overall body appearance into manageable, and hopefully more likable, parts.

On the following pages there are two written exercises which will help you learn how you feel about your body. You may find that this kind of mental looking glass is anxiety-producing. You may feel nervous; you may feel that there is altogether too much emphasis on physical beauty in this "thin is in" culture. You may be right about that. Nevertheless, we live in this culture and form opinions of our physical selves in part based on the feedback we get. You owe it to yourself to discover just how you feel about your body — your positive attributes as well as the body features you need to work on.

First, answer the ten questions on body image on page 87. What did you score? Remember, you'd be the rare overweight if you had a super-positive body image. So don't be unduly upset if you discover you have a poor one. At least, now you know what you are up against.

The next job, and a somewhat more pleasant one, is to separate your body into its many parts and take a look at each one individually. Total the number of "pleased" and "displeased" answers. Aren't you surprised at the number of body features that pleased you? So many times when we overweights look in the mirror and see nothing but fat, we are unnecessarily dooming ourselves to a totally negative body image when it is probably not true at all. For example, I knew a young woman who weighed close to 300 pounds but she had shiny, luxuriant honey-gold hair hanging to her waist. It was a crown, a veritable halo, and drew everybody's immediate attention whenever she entered a room; so much so that people, involuntarily, reached out to touch it. Yet, Sharon had such a negative body image of herself that she allowed the negativity to cancel out this extraordinary feature.

Notice, in particular, the "Pleased" checkmarks you made in the *Face* section of your Body Features Evaluation. Psychologists tell us that a positive face image can make all the difference in our self-esteem. It seems that people who are satisfied with their faces are just naturally more self-confident.

Remember too, when checking your Evaluation, that a woman's self-esteem is especially centered on a pretty face while a man's self-esteem relates not only to being handsome but also to having a muscular chest.

Have you been honest in your Evaluation? It is no crime to say, "Yes, I like my nose/mouth/hands." In fact, it is a crime *not* to recognize that you have some very attractive features. One survey showed that overweight females were pleased more often than displeased with body features, by an average margin of two-to-one! Yet these same women all scored a negative body image on the Body Image checklist. Be kinder to yourselves. Let go of a totally negative body image, especially since you now have proof that it really isn't true.

Body Prejudice

Here is a good point to remember. Body prejudice or body hatred can kill. Women, in particular, who loathe to touch their bodies can fail to give themselves monthly breast examinations, or may be too embarrassed to submit to professional examinations. Cancers can lurk in large breasts, say doctors, just as they attack small ones. And don't think a professional will let you off when you tell him or her that your breasts are too big to check. It's just plain not true. A large woman should follow these recommended steps.

1. Between the tenth and fourteenth day after beginning menstrual flow, stand in front of a mirror with your breasts exposed (no bra) and look for any month-to-month changes in the shape and size of your breasts, any pulling-in around the nipples, any discharge from the nipples or any scaling. Look at them with your arms down at your sides, then raise your arms over your head. Next lean forward and place your hands on your hips, tightening your chest and arm muscles by pressing inward.

2. Lie flat on your back with a pillow or towel folded under your shoulders and feel each breast. Use your left hand for your right breast and vice versa. Feel for any lumps that are hard and well-defined under your fingers, in other words, lumps that have a form. Feel from the bottom to top and from the nipple to the sides of the chest, paying special attention to the area between the breast and the armpit, and to the armpit itself.

After a few months, you will get to know how your breasts feel and you will recognize any change. If you feel a lump, contact your family doctor for an examination appointment. Although most lumps are not serious, you will want confirmation from a physician so that you can be at peace in your own mind. Nothing panics a woman as much as a suggestion of breast abnormality. The few minutes spent each month in self-examination are a small price to pay for freedom from panic.

If you have large or pendulous breasts because of a long-term weight problem, don't let that stop you from seeking expert help. "There are as many different kinds of breasts as there are women," a nurse-practitioner told me, "and most women from the age of child-bearing on certainly don't have 'movie star' breasts. Besides, nurses and physicians who examine dozens of breasts every day are only interested in what's in them or under them." It's not how big or small your breasts are; getting to know them is the point.

Overweight men, too, as well as women, must get over body prejudice because it can kill. Body hatred can lead to body avoidance and you will probably not give your body the attention or maintenance it needs. O.K., you may not be as crazy about the way your body is made as you could be, but don't *hate it to death!*

What's Really Behind Body Hate?

There is a basis for being ashamed and disgusted with our bodies that goes beyond our weight problems to centuries, even milleniums, of the Judeo-Christian notion that the body is inherently suspect. We aren't born with body-hate, but we soon pick it up from a "body disparaging society," as Emily Coleman and Betty Edwards call it in their marvelous book *Body Liberation.*

For instance, take these examples of western religious thought. "The whole man," said John Calvin, "from head to foot is drenched in a flood of wickedness so that no part has remained without sin and so everything which springs from him is counted as sin."

Adds Martin Luther, somewhat redundantly: "Our weakness lies not in our works but in our nature; our person, nature and entire being are corrupted through Adam's fall." From these (and other) savants the idea arose among our ancestors that the body and the soul were constantly at war with each other, just as were good and evil.

Women were thought to have bodies that caused bad things to happen, especially to unsuspecting men, who would be unable to control themselves at the sight of a bare, feminine ankle. To counteract this "effect," the female body was covered from head to toe, hidden under layers of petticoats and corseted *even at night.* A well-bred woman wouldn't consider meeting a guest with naked hands and many ate with fingerless mittens because they couldn't stand to be seen "barehanded."

We can laugh today, but are we really light years beyond the prudery of these recent progenitors of ours? Apparently not. "The twentieth century may have learned to shorten bathing suits;" says Stephen Kern in his book *Anatomy and Destiny: A Cultural History of the Human Body,* "it may have campaigned for sexual liberation, but it still has not fully come to terms with the human body."

When people are taught that the body is wicked, they cannot feel like whole people. To accept one's body, to love it, to protect it with the best health maintenance, that is the fulfillment of the holistic lifestyle.

It is true that many of us have freed ourselves from the worst of Victorian body hatred, in particular the younger generation, but we overweights have a distance to go in order to feel a true acceptance of our outer selves, regardless of our size.

As you start along the road to a happier body image, there are two things to remember.

1. Do have a realistic standard of good looks for your body. There was only one Marilyn Monroe and only one Arnold Schwarzenegger. If you have such an impossible ideal, you make certain you can never measure up.

2. Allow yourself as many simple sensory delights as possible, believing that it is right to experience pleasure through your body.

Getting in Touch with Your Body Senses

The following pages are devoted to body awareness exercises which produced some startling and positive insights for individuals in my Body Image workshops for overweights.

You can take the same awareness exercises yourself. Here's how. First you should try to get in touch with your body, as it is at this moment, through relaxation.

1. Choose a quiet room and close your eyes.

2. Get yourself there and in that place. Let go of what happened today or yesterday. Leave all the anxieties, apprehensions and stage fright behind you. (Yes, some people feel what amounts to stage fright when they attempt self-discovery.)

3. Now, notice your breathing. No, don't change it, just concentrate on the rise and fall of your abdomen and the flow of air through your nostrils.

4. Next get into your fantasy world. Don't direct it. Just let it happen. Remember fantasy is any mental activity that's not happening at this moment. Relaxed body presence is what you're after so don't be concerned with the right or wrong way to do this. There is no right or wrong way — only your way. And your way can tell you something about yourself.

5. Can you get in touch with anything outside you? The hum of a machine, maybe, or the song of a bird near the window can help you focus.

6. Can you sense things inside you? Don't try to analyze these feelings. Just recognize them.

Now that you are in a relaxed state, take a pen or pencil and piece of paper and make a "sensual" history of your body. Begin to write all the body sensations you've had, the things you have touched, felt, tasted, smelled or seen. Write as many body sensations as you can remember from your life, both pleasant and unpleasant. Again don't try to direct the sensations to come, just sit for a minute and let them come, ranging over different periods in your life.

Read the sample lists collected from workshop participants on pages 86 and 87. Two interesting conclusions can be drawn from the sampling I took. Although respondents were given permission to include both pleasant and unpleasant body-sense memories, the majority of sensations remembered were pleasant ones. Only a few of these sensual memories had to do with food or body-hate. Again, you will find that when you break down your body feelings into manageable size, there is more to the good than you realized.

Take a minute or two to read back over your own list at this point. Get better acquainted with the body that felt these sensations. Try to get a feel for your body and the things you have been through together. Now that you have taken a sensual inventory, you are ready to write a dialogue with your body in conversational form.

Such a dialogue is really a very special kind of talking on a deeper level — soul to soul — with your physical self. It is quite simple to do. Taking a fresh piece of paper and your pen or pencil, begin by saying something to your body and allowing your body to answer back. You may find your body saying things you never thought you'd hear. Maybe you will have things to blame your body for, or things your body will blame you for. Again, let it all flow and be as spontaneous as you can. Don't censor. Don't justify. Don't explain. Just let it flow.

Here are some sample dialogues from my self-image workshops for the overweight, which show a range of emotion, confrontation and acceptance.

Young, single woman, now thin after many years of overweight

Mind: Hi, Body. You seem sad. Are you tired?

Body: Yeah, I am — kind of distant you know, nonfeeling. Maybe I'm scared to talk to you.

Mind: You had some good sensations in your day, but some seem so long ago. That old you was always stuffed with food. you sure can have *that* awful feeling. It was pure hell and no escape.

Body: It's a fantastic free feeling being without all that fat.

Mind: I really feel that we are together at this moment.

Married woman in her thirties, thinner by thirty pounds but not quite at her natural weight

Mind: How are you, Body?

Body: I'm better than I've been for a long time. I feel prettier and stronger and thinner than I ever remember feeling. Mind, I wish you'd relax. I know you feel guilty because you put too much bread and sugar in me last night. Why don't you stop and think where we were a year ago? We've made fantastic progress. Be thankful for that and don't be so rough on us just because you goofed. I'll keep sending good strong signals to you whenever you put the wrong food into me. All you have to do is be aware of the messages and try to take it easy. We'll make it in time.

Mind: I believe you but I feel deprived sometimes — like when I go through all the hassle of baking and decorating cakes and not getting any. I always have to be on my guard because of you.

Middle-aged woman of uncertain weight

Body: Why do you persecute me so? Why are you so hard on me? You know I don't like being so cumbersome and uncomfortable. When will all this end?

Mind: I don't know. I realize how unhappy you are but I find disciplining you so difficult and I give in to your most unimportant and insignificant needs.

Body: Please do treat me more kindly. Try to love me as I should be loved. I
am not dirty.

Man in his twenties after sixty-pound weight loss

Mind: Hey Body, you've served me pretty well, and I want to thank you.

Body: You've done well by me, too — most of the time.

Mind: When did I let you down?

Body: When you put more fuel into me than I ever needed to keep going.

Mind: You know I'm really trying to stop that.

Body: You're doing better. I don't puff as much at the gym these days, and
my heart rate is better.

Mind: There are a lot of things I'd like to do with you, but I can't because
there's still too much of you.

Body: I know what one of those things is. You want me to get in bed with a
great female body.

Mind: Yeah, . . . !

Woman in early fifties with over 100-pound weight loss

Mind: We are in this thing together, Body. Are you going to let me down? Are
you going to last long enough to let me do all the things I want to do?

Body: It seems to me that's up to you. If you take care of me, I'm more than
willing to go along. You know I have a couple of weak spots, especially when it comes to food, but I think we can make it.

Mind: You know how impatient I am. I want to hurry and get it all done. I'm
so afraid time will run out on me.

Body: I know but surely you realize — wait a minute, you think you're smart
— I'll do a lot better if you give me the rest and care I want.

Mind: Say, did I detect a note of sarcasm there?

Body: You sure did. You think you're so smart and I'm supposed to go along
and serve you, Mind, and postpone getting my needs fulfilled.

Mind: I have to admit you are right. I'm afraid I mistrust you, though it always
seems to me that the more I slow down for you the more you want to
slow down.

Body: Wait a minute! Think about that again. You have been taking better
care of me and I haven't been slowing down. In fact, I've been doing
better. Right?

Mind: Right. I guess we both have been doing better. I seem to be learning to
treat you well and you have gotten lots more accomplished with less
effort.

Body: I'm glad you have enough sense to realize that I think we are a good
team if we each keep track of the other's needs.

Woman, late thirties, slightly overweight

Mind: I can think of lots of things to say to you, Body, but you better not
answer back after all you did to me. If it hadn't been for you, I would
have had the life I wanted, but, of course, I wouldn't be where or who I
am today. On the whole, I guess, I like where I am now, so I can't be
too angry with you. If I'd had a beautiful body instead of you, I'd have
gotten into a heap of trouble.

O.K. now you ask me anything you want to know, except why did I distort you like I did. I don't know the answer to that one and, perhaps you had better not talk to me. I don't want to hear anything you could possibly say.

GOD KNOWS, I tried to help you! I got the by-pass surgery to help you. You don't believe that? You'd better. I wanted you to have a chance, and I didn't trust myself to give it to you. I've always been ashamed of you. I couldn't stand to look at you or touch you or have anyone else touch you.

Woman in late forties, lost thirty-five pounds over past year

Mind: I've never felt comfortable with you. You were either too fat or not stacked or not shaped or, whatever, but — never what I wanted you to be.

Body: And what was that?

Mind: Thin and desirable, comfortable, well-dressed. You get the picture? No floppy breasts and big arms, no fat, wiggly thighs and spider veins, no belly and no teeth rotten from too much junk food.

Body: Enough! Enough!

Mind: Well, you asked for it.

Body: While we're on the subject, I never thought you treated *me* very well, either. Always the tight belts and tight bras, shoes that hurt and nylon stockings ending too soon that let my legs rub raw — and those fat arms in tight sleeves! What a sorry trick to play on me.

Notice how many different possibilities are contained within a mind-body dialogue. Some are true exchanges between equals, but in one the mind dominated and in another the body dominated. Some of the dialogues are angry, some pleading or poignant, some proud. The point is that there is no right or wrong dialogue, only the one that flows between your mind and body. If you attempt the dialogue again next week or next month, it will be different, sometimes quite different. Many of us overweights have deep emotions of anger, despair and distrust to work through. As we bring these emotions out onto paper, we then become ready to move forward to another facet of this ever-fascinating relationship between mind and body, and ever closer to the real integration between these far too often warring partners. Ultimately we will come to permanent weight loss.

In time, you will begin to see a real change in the way you think about your body and in the way you perceive your body visually. You will become more and more in tune with the numberless nuances of the relationship between your physical and mental self. You will be able, with practice, to focus your attention more specifically, rather than just on "the big, fat slob" image. Some researchers believe that with proper training, we could even focus on individual cells in our body. Finally, we would come to believe, as bioenergetics expert Stanley Keleman believes, that, "We do not *have* bodies, we *are* our bodies." In other words, there is no separation between our mental, emotional and physical selves.

What Will Body Awareness Do for You?

If you have been participating in the written and mental exercises in this chapter, you have learned some positive new things about yourself and your body. How can you use this changed attitude in your plan to lose weight? The answer is simple. Remember when you resist a part of yourself, like your body, you can become so involved in resistance that you are negative toward everything — your health, your diet, your whole life. Conversely, when you actively seek out the positive body image, you begin to resist your body messages less and less.

Work for new feelings about your body, then go with these new feelings as far as they will take you. Chances are they will take you as far as you will ever want to go.

Three Ways to Relax and Improve Your Body Image

1. "What is life for, if not to dance!" asked Zorba the Greek. Without realizing it, the lusty Zorba articulated a message for overweights.

There is no better way to *feel* the aliveness of your body than through movement to music. An entire modern dance therapy has grown up around what one psychologist called a "moving meditation." It's a way of discovering the calmness in your center (that you probably didn't know you had), and it releases a flow of creativity that focuses your mind and your body, helping to eliminate the space between them.

Read "Dance With Your Body," on page 89: then do it. Repeat this body-image exercise whenever you have problems with your physical self. Try to remember that in this dance you are not performing, not even for yourself, but dancing with your own body as a focus for self-awareness. Psychologists who use dance therapy in groups report they see dramatic changes faster than through "talk therapy" alone.

One of these, Dr. Robert Picker, says the only "should" connected with dance therapy is that one must be aware of the experience without judging it. In that way we learn to own our experiences, cease attempting to control or change them and simply allow ourselves to be who we are.

Ask yourself: How can I be all that is possible for me to be? You will find some of the healing answers in better body awareness.

2. It is not always convenient to use dance therapy when you need to enhance your body image. You may have a houseful of nosy people, who would go crazy if you locked a door and turned on dance music. These are the times when you may want to try deep muscle relaxation, a method in use for years in Europe. Here's how to do it:

a. Find a quiet place. Get comfortable, either on your back or in a sitting position. Close your eyes.

b. If you're right-handed, begin by tensing your right hand and telling it to feel heavy and warm. Continue with the rest of the right side of your body, moving up the arm to the shoulder and then down to the foot and up the leg to the thigh. Next, follow the same procedure on the left side of your body. (If you're left-handed, reverse the procedure.) Your arms, hands and legs should feel *relaxed, heavy* and *warm.* If they don't, repeat the technique and wait for these feelings. After some practice, your muscles will relax without tensing, just because you want them to.

c. Next, work on relaxing the muscles of your hips and let a wave of relaxation move from the abdomen to the chest. Do not tense these muscles; just tell them to feel *warm* and *heavy.* Your breathing will begin to slow. Watch for this change.

d. Now, move the relaxation wave up into the shoulders, neck, jaw and face muscles. Finish this exercise by telling your forehead to feel cool.

Ideally, you should practice this body awareness and relaxation drill twice daily for about 15 minutes, but that may not be possible with your busy schedule. Three minutes several times a day is better than not relaxing at all. You will find body relaxation particularly helpful about an hour before meals or prior to situations (perhaps, social) which you expect may prove stressful.

3. At times you can get a good awareness of your body through exercising some mental muscles. Try this:

a. Enter a relaxed physical state by resting in a comfortable chair with your feet elevated or by lying prone on your bed.

b. Close your eyes, allowing thoughts of self-love to flow through your head. If negative thoughts occur, say "no" under your breath very softly.

c. Imagine your body in its wholeness, floating on a calm blue sea under a clear blue sky. (Psychologists say that the color blue is the most restful in the spectrum.)

d. Become aware of your breath as you inhale and exhale slowly. Your breathing is natural as is your body. Follow each breath as it flows in and out of the body that gives you life.

e. Repeat the word "love" in your mind over and over as you inhale and exhale. Love is flowing to you and from you.

There are dozens of other ways to enhance your body awareness and to achieve a better body image than you have had in the past. The holistic movement incorporates the practices of most of the world's healing traditions to help people help themselves. Many more of these methods will be mentioned in succeeding chapters.

Self-massage

For obvious reasons, when we begin to become better acquainted with our bodies, we may experience some embarrassment. We probably will be shy about allowing others to manipulate our bodies in massage. At least we'll be shy at first. Many of us don't stay that way when we discover how wonderful our bodies can really feel after letting go of our negative self-image.

Did you know your skin is loaded with 50 receptors for every 100 square millimeters of skin? *It is made to feel.* Touch it. Touch is one of the most effective means of getting to know your own body in a positive way. Touching is a caring, healing form of self-acceptance. The "laying on of hands" has been an accepted form of healing since Biblical times, and this meaning has been extended to self-healing in the holistic movement. Self-massage relaxes your body, increases circulation and promotes a sense of well-being within you. It is a deeper form of communication between your mind and body.

Here is a simple self-massage you can give to yourself, to help you literally get in touch with and learn to know your living body. Choose a comfortable surface where you will be free to lie prone or sit up. A bed, sofa or heavily carpeted floor will do. Try to breathe calmly, maintaining a rhythm with the strokes of your hands. This combination of breathing and stroking will increase the deep relaxation you will feel.

Basic Self-massage

Toes:	Begin with your toes, the point most distant from your heart. Manipulate your toes by bending and pulling and working them around in circles.
Foot:	Move up your foot, using both hands to knead the ball and instep.
Ankle:	Hold your ankle with one hand and rotate your foot with the other.
Calf:	Rub your lower leg up and down, kneading the calf with both hands.
Thighs:	Grasp the skin on the outside of the thigh and rotate it over the muscles.
Abdomen:	Using first one hand and then the other gently stroke the abdomen in clockwise circles.
Chest:	Both men and women should massage their breasts using both hands, first in a clockwise motion then in the reverse.
Shoulders and arms:	Massage your shoulder in long strokes to the wrist, first down, then up. Do this many times for both shoulders.
Neck:	Stroke your neck with both hands, kneading the muscles at the base of the neck and top of the back as far as you can comfortably reach.
Face:	Gently tap the face all over with the tips of your fingers, alternately stroking with an upward motion.
Hands:	Do the same for the hands and fingers as you did for your feet and toes. Manipulate and rotate your fingers and knead the palms of your hands while stroking the backs of your hands toward your heart.

Just lie there quietly for a few minutes. You should have an almost euphoric, tingly feeling. This body-awareness will grow as you gain proficiency at relieving tension from knotted muscles; that is, if you are not, pardon the expression, rubbing yourself the wrong way. Remember, don't use a heavy stroke, and if your skin is chapped or dry, add some oil to your fingers as they move about your body. Gift yourself with the most pleasant experience you can, which brings us to a supremely self-pampering, indulgent massage you can give your body.

The Body Awareness Spa in Your Bathroom

Women, especially, will find self-massage in their bath a delightful way to become body conscious. It is sensual, delightful, soothing, calming, restorative and inexpensive. Your bathtub is much more than just a place where you cleanse your body. You can actually renew it and your sagging motivation as well. When you're feeling particularly deprived because of some "gooey" you've denied yourself, one of the best things you can give yourself (and certainly the lowest in calories) is a luxury bath. Why not? You deserve it.

Vital moisture, soothing warmth and a gentle motion make the simple ritual of taking a bath one of the most therapeutic things you can do for your body. Water is pleasurable and good. It's a tonic. You can steep all your senses, relax tired, sore muscles and become totally aware of every inch of your own body.

Pamper yourself. As you climb into your warm tub, have an array of bath accessories that would put a sultan's harem to shame. (They're not even expensive — about the price of one week's supply of cookies.) I like huge silk bath sponges, scented oils and bubble baths, a long-handled brush, a loofah scrubber for circulation and a bath pillow to loll on as the tub surf rolls in.

For the finest (and funnest) bath products write for the Caswell-Massey catalogue, 320 West 13th Street, New York, New York, 10014. Enclose $1 and postage.

Make the most of your body senses during your bathing times. Here are some hints for the perfect bath:

1. Bath water should never be hotter than your body temperature or you will tend to lose too much moisture.

2. Spoil yourself with a riot of fragrances.

3. Repeat the Basic Body Massage for at least ten minutes, while your body is submerged in silky, warm water.

4. Use a pumice stone to smooth any rough spots on your feet or hands, elbows or knees.

5. Dry with a heavy terry beach towel.

6. Use a skin moisturizer all over your body after your bath.

Men, and women too, who shower may want to follow the Basic Body Massage with a cool shower or give their capillaries a thrill with an alternating warm then cool spray.

Both men and women will want to try the following body massage with a towel, during or immediately after a shower or bath.

Basic Friction Massage

1. Choose a rough textured toweling.

2. Holding one end in your left hand and the other end in your right hand, begin to towel the upper back briskly with your head thrown back. This helps shorten the upper back muscles, straighten the neck and get rid of that fatty hump some women develop on the upper back.

3. Drop the towel to the lower back and massage, pulling the towel from side to side, first with one, then with the other hand.

4. Next, take a washcloth of the same textured material and apply a deeper friction rub, making small circular movements on the back of the neck, the upper arms, outer thighs and anywhere fat collects. It draws the blood to these areas, gets it circulating and cleans your skin by sloughing off dead skin cells.

5. Finally, stroke your skin with a light, warm oil (like baby oil) always moving firmly in the direction of the heart.

Learning to give your body the sense that you care about it will be easier than you think. As you progress in self-love, you will become more relaxed, less fearful of your body and far less prone to body-avoidance. Why don't you try it? Don't say it won't work until you've actually followed these instructions and become better acquainted with the outer you. It works, if you work at it.

The Other Side of Holism

The holistic mind-body dieting concept has a third component to its unity equation, and that component is the spiritual. Although this may be a *health* concept new to you, it is not so far-fetched when you broaden the scope of spiritual to include more than formal religion. You have a spiritual side to your holistic plan for permanent weight loss and good health if you incorporate any of the following in your daily life:

1. Love of God and His divine laws.
2. Love and respect for yourself and faith in self-healing.
3. Love of life and nature.
4. Love for your fellow human beings.
5. Belief in prayer or meditation.

As you read on, you will want to grow in one or more of these areas of spiritual holism to complete the picture of you breaking out of the fat cell where you have been trapped for so long. Think of the spiritual side of your program as an attempt to reach a higher self and then to form a unity between that self (ego or soul), your mind and your body. You were born with an integrated nature which fractured because of weight gain and stressful living, and now you are seeking to integrate yourself again. You are only reclaiming what is rightfully yours. An ancient Indian philosophy puts it this way:

> "I was one, I became many,
> and now I am One again."

The Whole You

One of the main concepts of the holistic healing movement is to concentrate on wellness as opposed to thinking of the body only when it's sick. In this chapter (and in earlier chapters as well), we've talked about some of the things that are "well" about you, that are good about you, that you can love about yourself without shame. We've talked about the unity of mind, body and spirit as a basis for a lifetime plan of weight losing and maintenance for your health's sake.

After discovering there are many body features you like, you will never again be able to think of yourself as *only* fat. You will have a more balanced estimate of just how you look. In this chapter you've dialogued with your body, and will continue this dialogue as one of the most natural things you do, so that never again will you be totally out of touch with your physical self. You are in training to be fair to yourself, and as a result you have a better-balanced body image and a far better chance of reaching the thinner body image you fervently desire — and staying there.

The bars on your fat cell are beginning now to bend and fall away, one by one. Isn't it about time?

The point of this book is to get beyond just plain dieting into a higher, inner, more integrated way of living. You may think that nothing is happening to you while you read, but your thinking patterns are subtly rearranging themselves. It will not be possible for you to return to your old patterns of self-blame, defeatism and negative body image.

In the following chapter, you will find out if that old myth about the unsexy fat man and woman is really true. Fair warning: you should prepare yourself for a great, big, sexy surprise.

Sample Sensual Inventories

Woman, 38

1. being held by a man
2. orgasm
3. hearing music
4. smelling pine needles
5. singing to myself
6. using my body in a sport and feeling "good fatigue"
7. feeling the terrible agony of carrying around too much fat
8. riding home in the car and leaning against mother
9. rocking my babies and feeling the round softness of their bodies against mine

Man, 32

1. that marvelous touch sensation when I hit a baseball, tennis ball or golf ball correctly
2. the smell of smoke
3. hiking through leaves
4. the sharp, ice-cold hurt of beer on my throat in summer
5. roll of kettle drums
6. eating ice from an ice truck
7. feeling tall
8. seeing the ocean for the first time
9. kissing
10. kicking my brother in the shins

Woman, 56

1. sitting on my father's lap
2. smelling Mom's home-baked bread
3. wetting my pants as I walked home from school in the third grade
4. holding my mother's hand when she died
5. touching a fish when I caught it

Woman, 35

1. eating pickles
2. soaking in a hot tub with good smelling bath salts
3. dancing
4. the smell of clothes on a line

5. the feel of tree bark on my skin
6. waking up after an operation and loving every cell of my body
7. getting drunk

Woman in her thirties
1. cashmere
2. snow
3. Estee Lauder perfume
4. spare ribs and kraut
5. riding a train
6. squeezing anything
7. the smell of coffee
8. falling off a merry-go-round
9. the taste of salt on my skin
10. when my hands feel soft
11. goose bumps

Do You Have a Negative Body Image?

1. I try to avoid full length mirrors and only seek those which reflect my head and shoulders.   Yes   No
2. I wear clothing of a style and color which will hide my extra pounds.   Yes   No
3. I will not allow a salesclerk to help me when trying on clothes.   Yes   No
4. When I look in the mirror, I feel bad about all the food I've eaten today.   Yes   No
5. I have often been self-conscious with people I am attracted to because of my body's appearance.   Yes   No
6. I never undress in front of my sex partner.   Yes   No
7. At a party, I will try to hang on to my coat or hold on to a pillow to cover my body jiggles.   Yes   No
8. I never exercise in public because of the way my body jiggles.   Yes   No
9. When I'm getting up from a soft sofa or deep chair, I do not like for people to watch my gracelessness.   Yes   No
10. I never swim at a public beach. Yes   No

If you answered yes: 1-3 times, you have some negative body image; 4-7 times, you have a negative body image; 8-10 times, you have a very negative body image.

Your Body Features Evaluation

	PLEASED	DISPLEASED
Face		
Complexion		
Ears		
Nose		
Mouth/lips		
Chin		
Teeth		
Eyes		
Upper Torso		
Neck		
Shoulders		
Chest (male)		
Chest hair (male)		
Breasts (female)		
Extremities		
Upper arms		
Hands		
Fingers		
Legs		
Upper thighs		
Feet		
Lower Torso		
Abdomen/stomach		
Buttocks		
Sexual Organs		
Vagina		
Penis/testicles		
Overall Appearance		
Height		
Weight		
Skin Tone		
Muscle Tone		
Posture		
Hair		

HOLISTIC LIFESTYLE CHANGE 6

During the next week, I will daily:

1. Dance with my body

2. Use either the Basic Body Massage or the Basic Friction Massage

3. Read one book on the holistic healing concept such as *Healing* by Dr. Jack LaPatra

4. At the end of the week, immediately after performing one of the basic body massages, I will dialogue with my body once again and compare it with the first dialogue I made.

Dance With Your Body

1. Go to a room where you have access to a record player and put on your favorite music. Try to have at least thirty uninterrupted minutes of music available.

1. Take off all your clothes. Set your body free of everything — glasses, shoes, watches — everything that would hamper movement. Then, dance.

3. All the space in the room is yours. Use it. Dance.

4. Allow spontaneity to flow. Do not dance against the music, but flow with it. In this way you will not lose energy, but gain it. Dance.

5. Forget your inhibitions. No one is looking and you are not being graded on your fox trot. Forget every step you ever learned. Arthur Murray prepared you to dance with others; this dance prepares you to be a good partner for yourself. Dance.

6. Do not look in a mirror. If there's one in the room, cover it over so that it will not distract you. This is not a confrontation; it is mind-body meditation. Dance.

7. As you dance, feel the suppleness of your muscles, feel the grace of your body, feel the intimacy you may never have felt for yourself before. Dance.

8. Never think of yourself as a weight while you dance. Think of yourself as free, lovable and attractive. Dance.

9. Think how blissful it is to let go, to set your body in motion without layers of constricting clothes and to feel your body in a stream of free-flowing energy. Dance.

10. Own your body. Have fun with it. Touch it. Dance away all tension, all dis-ease, all self-hate. Dance.

Chapter Seven

The Sexy You

If you ever doubt the connection between sex and food, watch the eating scene in the movie *Tom Jones* the next time it plays on the Late, Late Show, or remember that Casanova, no slouch as a lover, adored dropping raw oysters down a young lady's bodice and retrieving them with gustatorial glee. The erotic possibilities of food and eating are endless. Why then has the myth of arrested sexuality grown up around the overweight?

For years, some psychiatrists, starting with Freud, fostered the view that overweight, particularly in females, was based on the fear of sex. In other words, they promoted a theory that people gain weight because they want to hide their sexuality behind an armor of fat. This viewpoint has been almost universally accepted, especially by fat people. We overweights have been fed a steady diet of information which seemed to give us one choice: orgasm or chocolate bonbons.

New research refutes this old cliche, but it hasn't been given the same widespread attention that the Freudian concept received. It's about time you knew the truth.

Dr. Barbara Edelstein, author of the book *A Woman Doctor's Diet for Women* and a trained psychiatrist as well as a general practitioner, says she thinks the "fear of sex" theory is overdone by her fellow psychiatrists and even a "con." She states that she has found her patients relatively free of such neurotic tendencies.

Such conclusions can be easily supported when the old myth is brought face-to-face with Dr. William Shipman's work at Michael Reese Hospital in Chicago. Shipman chose 30 almost perfectly matched married couples. Only one difference existed. Fifteen of the wives were obese (more than 20 percent over their natural weight) and the other fifteen wives were of normal weight. Guess what the doctor found, much to his surprise, since he had thought to prove the opposite? The overweight women in the sampling not only had as much sex (two or three times a week) as their thin counterparts, but *wanted even more,* as opposed to the sexually satisfied thin wives. "These women," Shipman points out, "obviously aren't overeating *instead* of having sex; their craving for both food and sex exists simultaneously."

Researchers believe this study casts serious doubt on the widespread belief that many women become overweight to avoid sex, and that one of the problems accompanying obesity is lowered sex drive.

Dr. Abraham Friedman, a Florida obesity specialist, has come up with a novel twist on the old obesity vs. sex battle. He thinks that the overweight should substitute sex for food (instead of the other way around). "If you're still hungry after sex," he contends, "you haven't done it right." Although *he* doesn't say so, perhaps you should go back and do it over until you get it right, since each sex act uses 200 energy calories.

The other cross on the back of many fat women is the one labeled femininity. To be big in our culture is to be masculine, not feminine, so we are told. But is it?

Dutch doctor Frits deWaard believes that, in addition to ovarian hormone production, small estrogen factories in every cell of a woman produce part of the estrogen load. Since larger females have more cells than smaller females, doesn't it stand to reason that large women produce *more* female hormone? Strictly speaking, more female hormone circulating in your body makes you more, not less, feminine.

Nor does the argument rest there. The Harvard Medical School cites findings that women who have the greatest difficulty with weight consistently score higher on the femininity side of personality tests. Other studies in both the United States and Britain show larger-than-average women are characterized by a need to show affection, love of socializing and a more acute sensitivity to the feelings of others; traits which in this or any other culture are labeled "feminine."

Overweight men have the same problem, albeit to a lesser degree than women, in our "thin-is-where-it's-at" society. Although big can be masculine to a certain degree, too big, especially the development of fatty breast tissue, is considered feminine. Is that so!

Anne Scott Beller, in her book *Fat & Thin: The Natural History of Obesity*, cites two studies which show overweight fathers tend to have larger families than do thin fathers. She asks the question: Does fleshiness in males mean they could be *more* sensual?

By this time, you've begun to find your own answers, and realize what a double bind you've been caught in. All the talk about the lack of sensuality in the overweight has discouraged you from expressing your own and actually lessened your ability to lose weight. Fat people have been caught in another Catch-22 so prevalent in the dieting game: we are told on the one hand that we're not sexy if we aren't thin, and on the other that we stand a better chance of thinning if we are able to lead full, satisfying sex lives.

Set yourself straight on one thing. You *can* lead a full sexual life right now. From where you are. Whatever you weigh. Why? Because you are a sexy human being. *Very sexy.* You aren't hiding behind a barrier of fat. Your pounds are the too-solid indication that you are *a person of appetite,* a huge, vital appetite for life. You aren't just stimulated by the sight and smell of food, you can be enormously stimulated erotically and more sexually insatiable than thin people.

"Ordinarily heavy people," says Dr. Theodore Rubin, "are often very alive, and sensuous . . . Sex plays a large part in their lives . . . (They) have strong feelings and appetites that are often expressed with exuberance and abandon.

"Fat people are 'people people' and can both receive and give from and to other people."

Dr. Rubin lists among the sexy qualities of the overweight: zest, sensuality, sensitivity, expressiveness, enthusiasm, vitality, aliveness, strong feeling, involvement, responsiveness. In short, he describes people who express their humanity in such abundance as to be nearly overwhelming.

So why have you bought (if you did) the myth of the sexless overweight? Why, to paraphrase Mae West, did you make such a big issue over a little adipose tissue?

There is a simple answer to those questions. Because of society's prevailing attitude toward fat people, overweights *themselves* limit what they can be. We say, "I'm not supposed to feel sexy because I'm fat, so therefore I won't." We then begin to distrust our own nature and set in motion the wheels of self-hate and love-deprivation.

Kenneth Wachtel, writing on the social implications of overweight, thinks the general discrimination against fat people in thin America is partially sexual in nature. "The so-called beautiful people," he says, "use the mass media to project their own

'perfection.' The need to be considered 'in' leads directly to ridicule of those seen as excluded from the in group." Wachtel says
he questions such attitudes because they could serve as a mask
for some deep-seated fears on the part of "in" thins. Could it be
they fear that fat people are really highly sexed and, therefore,
competition?

As you have seen already in this chapter, Wachtel's suspicion
stands on solid ground. Be honest. The ridicule of fat sensuality by
thin America has led to your being ashamed and disgusted with
your body. Since the predominant aesthetic judges fat as unattrac-
tive, by society's standard a fat man is not a "real" man and a fat
woman is not a "real" woman. People imbued with these feelings
are going to have to work hard at viewing themselves as having
sexual rights.

Nobody is suggesting you may want to stay fat and sexy. Who
wouldn't rather be thin and sexy? But that's not the point. The
point is, as it has been throughout this book, that you have
precious little chance of being able to achieve permanent thinness
without a total lifestyle change. You cannot succeed in the weight-
losing game with a plan based on misery. You can succeed only
with a plan based on the victorious knowledge that you are a
beautiful, worthwhile human being — yes, and a sensual one, too.
You already own all the things you want to be. You cannot
become. YOU ARE. From this base of self-esteem and self-trust,
you can begin to make holistic lifestyle changes in the way you live
and, especially in the way you eat.

So there you are. Being overweight needn't affect your sex life,
if you don't *expect* it to.

The Fear of Sex Gone Wild

Let's get rid of one fat-making fear at the outset. Some overweights (and not just women, either) believe that should they
become thin they might not be able to restrain their sexuality. "I'm
afraid of what I might do," they chorus.

This is the direct result of postponing sexuality, of thinking
you're not good enough to have a sexual life now, as you are. No
wonder, with your appetites, you suspect you might go a little
overboard once you become thin.

Don't create such unnecessary anxiety for yourself. If you accept yourself as a sexual being today no matter what your size,
you'll be more able to handle your sexuality as a thin person. If

you feel comfortable and secure with the self you are now, you will not feel like a stranger to yourself just because your body has lost pounds.

Although this is a very real fear for many overweights, one diet club wit put the fear of sexual excess in perspective when she said: "I'm not worried about becoming thin and irresistible. I'm worried that I'll get thin — and still be resistible."

Body Image and Sex

Don't try to deny yourself that body image is important to your sex life. A positive body image contributes not only to self-esteem but also to a happy sex life. It is almost impossible to relate well to the opposite sex without the self-esteem a good body image brings. Both men and women who like their bodies have more sex, more partners and enjoy sex more than people with negative images. All these findings, certainly not surprising, were the result of the *Psychology Today* body image quiz.

Although it may be difficult to understand how your body image work in Chapter Six can influence your total lifestyle, it's best to continue working on it, rather than bemoaning the "beautiful people" syndrome of our current culture.

You may need to incorporate a routine of body awareness written exercises and massages into your daily life until they become second nature. This is especially necessary until you "own" the new physical body which is the aim of your holistic dieting. Once you have a slender body, your work won't be done — just changed. You will no longer need to spend your energy convincing yourself to love your physical self. You will spend the bulk of your energy convincing yourself that this new and slender you has really happened.

Until then, and even after, set aside some portion of your day, if only a few minutes, and devote yourself to yourself — to enhancing your body image and your sex life. Remember, the lack of self-love in your life leaves a curious sense of disembodied unrealness. Only with self-acceptance and self-love can you become *real* to yourself and able to truly give that self in lovemaking.

Getting in Touch with Your Sexual Self

Before you can reach the depths of your sexual self, you must discover who this sexual being really is, what sexual messages formed your makeup and what your sexual philosophy has come to be. That seems like a very large order, but, actually, you can gain great insight by spending a little time with your memory.

Get a pen or pencil and a piece of paper. Separate the paper into four different headings labeled: family, peers, society and religion. Then, under the heading, list the sexual messages (messages that formed your sexual image) that you received from each as a young person.

In my body image workshops for overweights, the final session was always devoted to pencil and paper confrontations with the individual's sexual identity. The following are some interesting messages members recalled.

Family Sex Messages

Mothers in my sampling were, as you might suppose, prone to give Victorian sex messages to their daughters, such as: "Nice girls don't do it," "Little boys are nasty," "Don't ask embarrassing questions," "Don't show your body," "You have a pretty face but if you don't lose weight you'll never catch a man," and "When you're married, you'll have to put a padlock on your nightgown." A minority of maternal sex messages were positive ones, such as: "It can be satisfying and fun," and "Women are just as hungry for it as men."

Fathers' messages to daughters in my workshops were for the most part suspicious and contained an added dimension of female accountability for male sex drives: "Don't turn boys on," "It's O.K. for boys and other girls, but not for my daughter," "Don't let anybody touch you, then you're 'damaged goods'," or "You can be touched, but don't touch the boy."

Both parents gave "fear of pregnancy" messages to their daughters.

The men in my workshops, of course, got different messages. The mothers in this sampling gave no spoken messages. Fathers and brothers were reported as having said: "Take it where you can get it," "You're too fat to get top flight stuff," and "Don't get caught."

It is not my intention here to enter the sex-role controversy. That society, and therefore our families and ourselves, has created a sexual double standard for men and women seems beyond question. If you want to know more about this problem and how it affects you, the reading list at the end of the chapter may help. The purpose of this chapter is to help you cope with your sexuality as a part of your total holistic dieting program.

What do you think the result of negative sex messages are for female-male relationships and marriage? What kind of messages did you receive from your family?

Peer Sex Messages

One workshop participant, a woman, thought all her adolescent peer messages had been lies. "We don't do anything wrong," they'd say, "but do you know what Mary did?"

The opposite (super-stud) peer messages among boys was, "I'm having sex all the time, and you're not!"

Both sexes received spoken messages that they were unsexy because they were fat.

Again, peers, like parents, gave out "fear of pregnancy" sex messages to each other.

What peer messages influenced your sex life most?

Society Sex Messages

"Real love is being captured and carried off by a pirate," said one Hollywood-struck woman. Said another, "Hollywood showed me that only beautiful, thin people can love and have sex."

Society (as reported by workshop members) valued virginity in women and Don Juanism in men until marriage, according to "messages" participants picked up from their culture. Remember not all messages are spoken. Some are implied by behavior and custom.

What implied messages did you receive from your culture?

Religious Sex Messages

Strangely, the makeup of my body image/sex workshops seemed to be equally divided between Catholics and Baptists, which does not imply that people of these religions are more troubled (or fatter) than others, just that the religious factor in any group of over-weights is unpredictable. In any event, see if you can relate any of the sex messages these people received with those on your own list.

One woman in her late thirties remembered: "The nuns at school implied sex was dirty, except to have a child. They indicated that, other than for procreation, there was no earthly reason for it. They always had a story of a woman saint who died horribly rather than be sexually violated.

A man received this message from a priest: "Men have no control. Women do."

Another woman got these sex attitude messages: "I remember asking a Sister what a word meant and she was shocked that I would ever have heard it."

"My church's teaching was that sex was a sin unless in marriage, then I was to do whatever my husband wanted to do as long as the seed was deposited in the proper receptacle.

"I was also taught not to be impure (masturbate) with myself."

One Baptist woman remembered: "I really thought the church was telling me that wearing lipstick, going to movies and dancing were more sinful than sex. I remember one of the jokes we told on ourselves was: Question: Why don't Baptist couples have sex standing up? Answer: Because the preacher might think that they're dancing?"

A male Baptist got this message: "Sex is good when you're married. Before that, play a lot of sports."

A second woman was told dating more than one boy at a time was sinful.

It is interesting to note that few of these sexual messages concerned weight; most had to do with prevailing female-male sexual custom. Nevertheless, it will come as no news to you, especially if you were a fat young person, that your adolescent size played a very great role in how you feel about yourself today. There is every possibility that an absence of sexual acceptance during crucial adolescent years makes it difficult for you to explore and share the sexual experience.

How would you like to behave as a fully functioning sexual human being? One more written exercise will help you to clarify your feelings about your own sexuality and give you a target at which to aim.

Reread your page of the written sexual messages you received as a young person. How would you change the negative messages into positive ones? Now take up your trusty pen or pencil and a fresh sheet of white paper; place on top the words Positive Sexual Messages to Myself and begin to write. Here are some workshop examples.

Woman #1: Sex is to be enjoyed! It is a pleasure, not a duty. I can engage in sex and relish it no matter how fat or thin I am or my partner is.

Woman #2: I acknowledge that sex is O.K. for me. I feel myself getting less and less inhibited. I realize that even though I am very obese, there are still men who are attracted to me.

Woman #3: I *can* enjoy sex at any weight and I plan to take advantage of any opportunity that comes my way. It's possible to be psychologically normal and still be super sexy.

Woman #4: I am lovable and desirable. It is all right for me to experiment to see what I am capable of doing, but I should stop short (if possible) of an orgy.

Male #1: Sex is good. It's fantastic! I'm thin now and I have closer relationships with many women. I like to have sex with a lot of women. I'd get too involved and anxious with just one. Someday I hope I can change that.

Woman #5: I'm going to try it with the light on tonight because I'm sexy no matter what my size is. I may even follow my instincts and be aggressive with my husband.

You get the idea. Give yourself a positive ideal to live up to. Open yourself to the "pleasurable lifestyle" as clinical psychologist Stella Resnick calls it. Indeed, Dr. Resnick suggests we actively pursue pleasure. No, don't be afraid of it. You, of all people, deserve more pleasure in your life. "People who live a pleasurable lifestyle," says Dr. Resnick, "are considered self-indulgent, maybe selfish and narcissistic, even (God forbid) hedonistic. What's wrong with a little enlightened hedonism? I think it's good for us."

Deprivation, not overindulgence, breeds greed, says the doctor. But if you feel nourished and satisfied, you want to share your good feelings and you have more to give. The process of becoming a more fulfilled, more turned-on person is a process of self-nourishment — not with cookies but with food for the spirit.

The Sensuous Dieter

The problem with too many overweights, both men and women, is that they have turned off their come-on. It didn't happen overnight or for any one reason. Perhaps you were rejected very early in life because your parents couldn't accept a fat child in their family. Perhaps you were accepted and loved by your family but rejected by someone else as you grew up or even after you became an adult. But the illogical and awful result for us overweights is that once rejected by another, we turn around and reject our own sexual identity. Not even the worst criminal is subjected to double jeopardy, but that is exactly what fat people do to themselves. We accept double punishment, first from the rejecter and then from ourselves. When you stop to think about it, isn't that tragic? Would we ever kick a friend who was already down, bruised and battered? Of course not, but that's not the end of the punishment we give ourselves for the horrible crime of being fat. We gradually train ourselves to turn off our sensuality. It's safer, we think, to present ourselves to the world as having no sexual needs at all. After a few years of such torture, we can actually begin to believe that we have no sexual desire. The truth is that we have deliberately banked the fires of passion; we have literally exiled our sexual selves to an emotional Siberia.

Today you love yourself and are working out a holistic plan to heal yourself, including healing the sensual you. But you didn't turn your sexuality off in a day and it will take time to make friends with that part of yourself again, to develop the ability to be intimate. Why not try these first simple steps?

Learning About Yourself (And Others) Through Touch

You are going to have to get to know your living body. Some of the self-massage techniques in the last chapter have helped you accept and love yourself as you are. You have actually felt your full-figured curves and contours and pointed out to yourself the features you like. Keep accentuating that positive.

Did you know that touch is a more basic need than sex? Dr. Harry Harlow took some infant monkeys away from their mothers and let them grow up without the cuddling and fondling they needed. Some of the monkeys developed destructive behaviors, some even died, wasting away for want of touching.

There comes a time when self-touching can naturally give way to touching by others. You may want to begin practicing some of the massage techniques you've learned with a partner. Slowly, cautiously you can open the door to a wider touching experience. When you are ready, you can discover a new dimension not just in your own body, but in your partner's as well.

Remember, you must keep it positive. As you stroke yourself or your partner, tell yourself: "How pretty this is," "How good this skin feels." As you repeat self-massage and mutual massage, those old critical thoughts will naturally be replaced with enhanced self-esteem. When you begin losing weight, touching will give you added incentive to continue.

Gradually you will lose anxiety, the same anxiety that caused you to turn your sensuality off in the first place. It is imperative that you do. The ability to communicate sexually depends on being as free as possible from anxiety.

Super-sensualize Yourself

Being sensual hasn't a thing to do with wearing a size five dress or having well-developed biceps. What is sensuality all about? You can easily spot it; it's that special quality of excitement that a man or woman imparts to others. First of all, sensuous overweights learn to find themselves exciting. They expose their senses to life's experiences. They show a real self-pride in every movement and in a well-modulated laugh and voice.

The sensuous overweight doesn't spend life in one long trek from bedroom to bedroom, collecting sexual trophies. Although your appetites for sexual experience are easily aroused, lovemaking is the result of your wish to share with another your love for your own sensual core. "The ability to share oneself," says Dr. William P. Angers, "is an integral part of sensuousness." Each act of giving, the psychologist goes on, has a dual effect: it reinforces your own sensuous self and tells your partner that you are sensitive to his or her needs.

Vital to your sensuous self is your ability to develop the totality of self, physically, mentally and spiritually. Have you ever admired the sensuality of someone who literally had to drag his or her body through life, who was mentally sluggish or emotionally overwrought? Probably not. That kind of poor self-image doesn't attract. *Other people are attracted to people who attract themselves, who genuinely love their real selves.*

You may find this hard to swallow, but one of the best sensualizing experiences is to drain every bit of pleasure from the taste of food. That's right. The Super-sensuous Overweight finds pleasure by truly tasting food. Too often we chew and gobble automatically without really tasting. If you do this, you are missing an opportunity to savor the juices and flavor of each bite; you are not allowing your taste buds time to enjoy to the fullest what you eat. If you practice eating sensually you will gain in two ways, by enhancing your ability to excite your taste sense and by slowing down the eating process. It's a simple equation — the more you savor the slower you eat, the slower you eat the fewer calories you take in and the more weight you lose.

You can carry sensual eating right out of the dining room to the bedroom. Carole Altman, in her book *You Can Be Your Own Sex Therapist* says that your highly sensitized taste buds can add a new dimension to lovemaking. Why not mix the taste of a favorite food with the taste of your mate or favorite sex partner? Try eating salad on your partner's stomach, she suggests for openers, and then proceed (without utensils, of course) through the entire meal, eating from various parts of your partner's body. Could the overweight lover's body with its generous nooks and hollows be especially adaptable for this erotic diet? You'll never know unless you *try it.*

The above sensuality exercise is a good example of the playful component in most truly sensual people. They take joy in experiencing for the experience alone. They touch often and can come close to being embarrassingly open. You can cultivate this sense of the joy of touching in your everyday life. Reach out to people. Take them by the arm, shake their hand, hug them. All of these gestures say "I like you" loud and clear. The ability to be a super sensuous overweight doesn't start in bed. It starts with a demonstration of affection all day long. You'll never know if it works unless you *practice it.*

Dr. Angers sums up the heart of sensuousness as being a passion for living, a feast of experience and a joy in sharing. Super sensuality is being fully aware of all your sensations, the exciting pleasures of touch, sight, sound, smell and taste that come to you each day. Remember the sensual memory inventory you took in Chapter Five? Take another one of the present day and, by comparing the two lists, see if you are not using your sense-abilities better than you were, just because you are more aware.

Ease into Sensuality

If you've been denying your own sensual appetites for years, don't try to blossom in an hour. Go courting. Court your sensual self with some well-thought-out moves.

1. *Learn to know your own needs, likes and dislikes and desires.* You don't enhance your sensual self if you hold your needs inside. Communicate your desires to your partner. Communication can be a great turn-on, but it also means risking rejection. This is something we overweights haven't tolerated very well in the past. So we must find ways to accept rejection. After all, no one, fat or thin, is accepted 100 percent of the time. It may be a signal that your

partner is in a "mood," or that he or she is unwilling to risk intimacy at that moment. It is not a rejection of *you*. Back in 1963, long before the human potential movement had a name, Laura Huxley wrote a gem of a little book called *You Are Not The Target*. If you are having trouble tolerating rejection and it interferes with your sensual life, get this book and read it.

2. *Learn to trust your body, your instincts and your own sensuality.* Out of your trust for yourself will grow a trust of your partner, without which there is no true sexual sharing. Trusting the other person makes it easier to expose your own sexual desires and increases the closeness you feel for your mate or sexual partner. Of course, even the closest relationship contains an element of privacy. There is no such thing as total sharing, but the more you can each share with the other, the more intimate your partnership can become.

Don't forget that not all relationships work out. When they don't, we should take some time to reassess what went wrong. This is *not* the time to put ourselves down, however, by heaping blame on ourselves and accepting total responsibility. That's not honest evaluation; that's our old enemy double jeopardy again. On the other hand, don't place all blame on the other person. That is a sure road to thinking "everybody's out to get me." That attitude makes honest relationships impossible because we will keep a large part of ourselves in isolation to avoid a big hurt.

We can't know ourselves or anyone else completely, but the more we learn, the more we will be willing to risk. That is what makes really sensuous relationships possible — even probable.

Fat people can be attractive and sensual. Are you hearing that message? Developing the sensual aspect of your mind and body will bring about a more perfect holistic union, diminishing the distance caused by living in a thin chauvinistic world. The "beautiful people" do not have a monopoly on love and sensual satisfactions. Isn't it silly to expect to hide your body in the dark, and deny your sensuality until you lose weight, and then to expect a sexual self to jump into being full-blown? You bet it is. Expressing your sensuality *while* you are losing weight (or even if you are on a plateau) is not only your right but an absolutely integral part of a holistic healing lifestyle. Don't forget that you are making a total lifestyle assault on obesity. You are:

• not blaming yourself for becoming overweight in the past, but you have decided to take responsibility for your health today.

• learning as much as you can about overweight because knowledge is a tool you can use for total living.

• becoming interested in nutrition, and, in particular, making decisions about what place refined sugar has in your diet.

• more positively assertive because you respect yourself too much to take thin chauvinistic abuse from an individual, society or even yourself.

• learning more about your wonderful body so that you can free it from its self-imposed fat cell.

You should be proud of yourself. That's a great deal to absorb and a great change to make in the way you live. You're going to find that even though change in anybody's life tends to be anxiety-producing in a sense, these changes, changes which emphasize the inseparability of mind, body and spirit, are healing the disease of obesity. But cure isn't enough for the holistic life. Healing, to be holistic in its nature, must incorporate growth, and you are seeing plenty of that in your changing life. Life for you has expanded. Your compulsion to fulfill the Earth Mother's cellular prophecy is self-limiting if you are following the precepts of holistic health. All the negatives will be left behind — for good.

Lovers Who Think "Big"

Lina Wertmuller, the famous Italian director, uses overweight actors in her movies because she says that she admires the full figure "for its soft external lines, for its rhythms that relate to nature and the life force, but that are indeed still dark and hidden and primordially mysterious." There's certainly nothing unsexy in Wertmuller's view of the overweight, nor in Dyan Cannon's. The former wife of slender movie idol Cary Grant states flatly (or roundly): "Fat men turn me on sexually."

Another thin woman reports she prefers her lovable fat boy-friend because thin men are "more into themselves — you know, stuck-up."

And it's not just women who like big men. Men like overweight women sexually. What is it, precisely, that some men see in fat women? One admirer claims that overweight females are less inhibited in bed. "There's a natural tendency to be more experimental, more versatile. You end up relating to more of her body than you would if she were thin."

Fat women think that men who admire (their) figures are superior lovers. "They take more time to caress, kiss and pinch," says Melanie. "He's usually much more into the flesh, the softness of it."

Writer David Haldane says his own research reveals that the majority of men who like fat women are "breast men" and simply find overweight women to be the best endowed. "There's something warm and comforting about the curves of a woman's body," says William Fabrey, the not-so-fat president of the National Association to Aid Fat Americans (see Chapter Ten for more about this group). "You can't possibly find a straight line on a fat woman."

Both male and female fat admirers claim that overweights make great lovers, not only because they try so hard to please partners, but because they have repressed their sexuality for so long that when they do let go, a dammed-up flood of sexuality breaks loose.

What's the point, if I'd rather be thin, you may well ask? Just this. Most of us overweights postpone sex, buying new clothes, finding a better job — everything, until we are thin enough to "deserve" them. Have you ever stopped to think that postponing life may be the very reason why so few of us ever get thin permanently? It is difficult, if not impossible, to work for yourself while in a state of misery and total deprivation. To lose weight, we will have to eat less, that's true, but do we have to live less? The answer is a resounding NO! Turn on your sexuality, allow your repressed appetites to be satisfied. Yes, those same appetites that made you fat in the first place can now be an important part of your lifestyle change.

Sex as Exercise

You will be reading more about overall body exercise in Chapter Eleven, but this seems to be a good time to talk about sex as exercise. Have you ever thought that sex has all the requirements of good sport? "It can be played year 'round," agrees weight expert and author, Dr. Neil Solomon. "It works best with another person. You don't need a large playing field or special equipment. You move every muscle in your body, depending on your degree of proficiency and, like all good sports, practice makes perfect."

Is the good doctor trying to tell us in a roundabout way that sex is good for weight loss? Another weight expert, Dr. Abraham I. Friedman, in his provocatively titled *How Sex Can Keep You Slim*, comes right out and boldly states that a single sexual session can use up 200 calories or more in addition to exercising and firming buttock, pelvic and abdominal muscles used in the sex act. "Make love, not fat," says Friedman who thinks the most frequent cause of emotional overeating stems from sexual problems and frustrations.

Absolutely right, agrees Dr. G. Scott Jennings whose sex therapy practice is devoted to helping overweight women release pent-up sexuality. "Whenever I find a woman overeating or even on a weight-losing plateau, I look for sexual frustration," says the doctor. "I find many of my patients have a high sex drive which could lead to one or more orgasms each day."

Dr. Jennings uses a number of methods to help the overweight and sexually thwarted female turn from food to sex for real satisfaction. He suggests:

1. Overweight women should make attempts through reading or consulting a sex-therapist, if necessary, to feel more at ease with their high sex drive.

2. Overweight women should try to become more aggressive sex partners.

3. Overweight women should be comfortable about stimulating their clitoris during intercourse if they need to.

What about masturbation? More and more men and women, as well as physicians, admit that it can teach you about your own sexual responses, and be a physical release technique. (Feminists even claim masturbation is lovemaking with the one you trust best, or at the least, is an alternative form of sexual expression.) If you are interested in learning more about this style of individual erotic play, in its more modern noncondemnatory aspects, read *Liberating Masturbation* by Betty Dodson, who writes the most upbeat work on the subject. (Remember to cut your calculation of caloric expenditure by half, to 100 calories when alone!)

It's no secret (or joke) that an active sexual life, particularly for the female, demands a supple, responsive body, a body which can perform with ease the Leg Stretch and the Tummy Tilt. No, these aren't two new rock and roll dances, but two sexercises to help you get into shape for your new more sensual lifestyle. And, best of all, they will only take three minutes of your busy day.

The Leg Stretch: Sit on the floor with your legs extended as far apart as possible. Lean over as far as you can and grasp as far down your leg working toward the day you can grasp your ankle. Hold this for a count of ten and then repeat on the other leg.

106

The Tummy Tilt: Lie on the floor, knees somewhat bent, feet planted firmly but slightly apart. Now lift off the floor, tilting your tummy, but keeping your back as straight as possible. This will work your buttocks and pelvis. Repeat the exercise, gradually bending your knees in an even greater angle so that more pull is felt in the tummy and pelvic region. Do this exercise for two minutes every day.

Why not add these sexercises to your regular self-massage routine? Now, you are ready for the new, sexy you. Get set. Go!

Satisfying Sex for the Overweight

If you have decided not to wait for the perfect figure before you release your abundant sexual appetites (since sexual activity is a way of insuring you'll have that thinner, healthier figure), then it's time to talk about special techniques which will enhance your lovemaking. Of course sexual technique is not the end-all of satisfying sex. It can be the kiss of death, if that's all there is to it. You will want to remember to be warm, loving, helping if you plan to be a skillful lover and gain and give maximum enjoyment. Sex, as one psychologist observed, can take on the quality of an improvised dance, changing rhythms, movement patterns, alternating leader and follower.

The two basic positions, man-dominant or woman-dominant may not supply you with "fancy fornication" as Marvin Grosswirth calls it, but these are two comfortable coital positions for the overweight that work well for most.

Man-Dominant: The man lies on top of the woman (supporting his weight with his elbows or hands). The woman, with legs spread apart lies upon a pillow to elevate the pelvis and provide easy entry for the penis. The woman can clasp her legs around the man's waist or even his shoulders if she is supple enough.

Woman-Dominant: One of the most satisfying positions for overweights is when the woman squats (or sits) over the prone man and guides his penis into her vagina. She can support her own weight or gradually lower herself against him. This position allows for the most complete freedom of movement, permitting stroking and caressing of practically the entire body for both partners.

If mates are King and Queen-sized, two other coital positions can be used for variety.

Rear Entry: The woman either kneels on the bed (or stands bent over) so that her buttocks are elevated. By kneeling (or standing) behind, the man can readily enter her.

Man Lying, Woman Standing: The man lies at the edge of the bed with his feet firmly on the floor. The woman, standing astride the man, guides his penis into her vagina. This has the same caressing advantages as the woman-dominant position, with the added advantage that no weight need be brought to bear on either partner.

Overweight sex mates can find (as do thin partners) that extravaginal coitus provides added variety to relationships. Stimulation by hand, tongue or mouth can be truly satisfying if religious or other prohibitions don't block their performance. Perhaps the most important thing to remember is that loving, sexual acts are never silent, dull or monotonous. Consummation is the culmination of special caresses by both partners surrounded by feelings of joy and warmth.

As you lose weight, you may want to expand your coital repertoire by taking a look at some of the 2,000-year-old literature on the subject such as the *Kama-Sutra* or the *Orissan* manual. On the other hand, you may find, at any weight, that slight (but inventive) variations on the positions outlined here are truly satisfying, unless, that is, you blossom into a circus contortionist or an Olympic gold-medal athlete.

A few final suggestions:

1. It makes sense to come to the love bed clean and well-groomed. Nothing is more a turn-off than body odor. (Sweat is no more masculine than it is feminine.) But remember that just because you're overweight, you're not automatically more prone to dirty skin, greasy hair or soiled fingernails. Despite the popular picture of the unkempt, slovenly fat person, Dr. Marvin Schroeder, a noted California surgeon, says his overweight patients are the "cleanest" he has, a situation that surprised him.

2. Since the sex act itself is not necessarily hampered by too many pounds, you can concentrate your energies on your attitude. You have every right to indulge your sexual appetites if *you think you have.*

3. It is just plain smart to avoid overeating right before sexual relations. Nothing detracts from sensual feelings so completely as the feel of another body lying athwart peanut butter sandwiches and cherry pie a la mode. To paraphrase Shakespeare, "Much food . . . takes away performance."

4. If you're dieting, don't overdo your intake of diet sodas. Carbonated bloat is also a sensuality wipe out.

5. Don't rush. You are a sense-able human being. Take time to enjoy the whole range of your senses — sights, tastes, sounds, smells and touches. Then too, on the practical side, the longer you take, the more calories you expend.

6. Avoid love-killing things, such as putting yourself down to your lover, being unwilling to experiment or being unwilling to take responsibility for your own pleasure.

Sex and Your Holistic Living Plan

Sex is an experience that can fill the mind-body-spirit needs of your holistic plan to lose weight permanently. With your five senses fully invoked you are practicing holism. When you breathe and love and stroke, you experience a merging of mind-body-spirit that is rather like exploring the self and becoming even more connected. You learn that you can provide *yourself* with happiness.

The heightened senses of sexuality help you to "listen" to yourself and be truly self-aware. The mysterious, the unknown, the future will not threaten you, if you *listen*. You will not be wary of your own past behavior, and will be able to rely fully on your own capabilities. You will learn what inner directions to follow, rather than blindly following the dictates of an often unthinking society. You will be better able, through listening, to make your own decisions, and maintain those points of view.

You may not be fully aware of it yet, but your mind is clearing and your deepest inner self is moving from a disharmony with life to a marvelous, sympathetic harmony. Your whole being is tingling with aliveness and the sure knowledge that, in time, you will heal yourself of the physical, mental and social effects of overweight. You are, at long last, becoming free from fear. You are saying to yourself, "I will have a whole, slender, healthy body some day, but I have the right to live and to love as I am now."

This week:

1. I will allow my sexual fantasies to develop where they will.

2. I will work to make my "love muscles" more flexible.

3. I will turn on my come-on and give out the message that I am a sexual being regardless of my size.

4. I will write a second set of *Positive Sexual Messages to Myself* and compare it with the first for growth.

5. I will tell myself every day that I am sensual and sexy, in other words a "real" woman or man.

6. I will touch (hug, shake hands, etc.) every person I meet.

Suggested Reading List

Altman, Carole. *You Can Be Your Own Sex Therapist,* Berkley/Putnam, New York, 1976.

Friedman, Abraham I., M.D. *How Sex Can Keep You Slim,* Prentice Hall, New Jersey, 1972.

Scheimann, Eugene, M.D. with Paul G. Neimark. *Sex and the Overweight Woman,* Signet, New York, 1972.

Chapter Eight

Choosing the Right Doctor

"Each patient carries his own doctor inside him."
— Albert Schweitzer, M.D.

Like a holy litany, the words "See your Doctor!" echo through dietdom's good books. Indeed, friends, family and even casual advisors chant the same phrase as if it were a sacred mantra for the overweight. Are they right? Yes. And no. See the *right* doctor, by all means, but just any doctor won't do for today's unashamed overweights. The question is: How you do find Dr. Right? That is what this chapter will show you, plus alerting you to your medical (and health) rights so that you won't stub your toe against the deep-seated prejudice some doctors have against the too fat.

How Could Doctors Be Prejudiced?

"Doctors are no more immune than anyone else to the influences of propaganda," says Theodore Rubin, M.D. "They are inevitably influenced as much by cultural pressures, conventions and styles."

There you have it from the doctor's mouth. And from research at Duke University, we learn that even pre-med students, when asked to describe fat people, responded with such adjectives as "disgusting" and "weak."

There seems to be no way that overweights can change (at least for a while) the way some doctors feel about treating us. Hippocratic oath or no, many overweights represent, as do alcoholics, visible records of a doctor's failure to cure. In other words, we don't always become walking advertisements for their skills. In such cases, some doctors would rather we didn't bring our health business to them. And that's probably all to the good.

On the face of it there seems to be two standard, if not too helpful, approaches by a fat-prejudiced doctor to his or her overweight patient. One, he ignores your weight problem (the Non-Recognition Syndrome) in a kind of updated version of *The Emperor's New Clothes* (he pretends your fat is invisible); or two, he treats nothing but your weight problem (the Over-Reaction Syndrome), ignoring other symptoms, often with some verbal abuse and total lack of understanding.

A recent report from Johns Hopkins Hospital states that 25 percent of doctors treating overweight patients chose to ignore their patients' fat. Although no studies have been done, a far greater percentage, according to accounts from overweight patients, are more prone to over-recognition than nonrecognition.

"You are just as healthy as an old cow," one jovial (if somewhat insensitive) obstetrician told a woman, reducing her humanity and her femininity to nil in one stroke.

"Your husband must really be turned off," commented another physician during a routine physical, in an unsolicited sexual evaluation. In fact, the woman's sex life was quite good.

Another woman reported that a doctor had laughed at her body during a childhood examination, laughter that she never forgot.

During one self-image workshop for the overweight, participants divided the contemptuous or prejudiced doctor's treatment into the following four types:

1. *The Hollywood Cure* — Doctors, most often men and subject to our culture's ideas about beauty and thinness, think they are appealing to a woman's femininity when they say, "You have such a pretty face, but you must lose weight." In truth, the doctor is negating the woman's femininity by telling her that no matter how pretty her face is, it's her body that really counts.

2. *Disgust Treatment* — Overweights report that doctors who say, "Go home, and look at yourself in the mirror," imply that the sight is so disgusting it will automatically cause the patient to lose weight. Chances are this sneering treatment will only subtract from the patient's already low self-esteem, making him or her even less likely to lose weight.

3. *Pontius Pilate Prescription* — "You're wasting my time," this physician says to the unsuccessful overweight, in effect washing his hands of further responsibility.

4. *Threat Therapy* — "Diet or die!" is the grim threat dieters face when doctors think scaring their patients to death will force them to solve the frightening problem about which they are consulting him in the first place.

IF ANY DOCTOR YOU CONSULT FOR HELP WITH YOUR WEIGHT PROBLEM USES ANY OF THESE DUBIOUS TECHNIQUES, IMMEDIATELY DISMISS HIM OR HER AS YOUR PHYSICIAN.

Dr. Right, when you find this physician, will be supportive, optimistic and have a nonthreatening attitude. Questions will be gentle, never uncaring. *Dr. Right* will never ignore the same symptoms that earn a thin person medication while giving you a diet sheet. The unprejudiced physician knows that the tragic consequence of biased treatment is that far too many fat people avoid going to the doctor at all costs. Not wishing to suffer humiliation and embarrassment, they let medical problems go undiagnosed and untreated, sometimes with fatal results.

You have the right to the best medical care no matter what your size. You have the right to be treated for the head cold, ingrown toenail or skin rash for which you go to the doctor's office. To have every symptom from infected warts to vaginal discharge dismissed as another result of your weight problem is to deny you equal medical care with the thin population. *That is another fat discrimination you don't have to take anymore.* After all, we hire doctors provide a service. They are neither gods nor "daddies," even though they usually assume the parental role. It's your money. You can hire or fire any doctor any time you aren't getting the care you want. You are in control of your own health.

Looking for Dr. Right

Now that you've decided to find just the right doctor for you, someone who will treat you with respect as an adult, you will want to begin your search in a logical way.

Too many times, we overweights take pot luck when it comes to the medical help we need. We'll settle for the family doctor, who may be perfect for the kids or for other family members, but is not helpful or understanding of our weight problem. We overweights should choose a doctor with the same care an accused felon chooses a lawyer. Our lives may depend on it!

One of the best ways to find a competent, unprejudiced doctor is by word of mouth. In this case, good news travels fast, so listen when members of your diet group or your overweight friends talk about their physicians. Question them about details of behavior and decide whether you would like to have a get-acquainted appointment. Failing a personal recommendation, call the county medical society and ask if there are any bariatricians (doctors who specialize in weight reduction) on their roster.

When you find a physician you would like to consult, be straightforward with him or her. You've probably had bad experiences with doctors before, but don't walk in with a chip on your shoulder. While it's true that certified bullies can wear white coats, some excellent human beings can wear them as well. Give the relationship a chance.

The Treatment's the Trick

You are not asking any physician for miracles, but you are asking for good treatment. Here is what you have a right to expect. Don't accept anything less.

1.   Never accept as adequate the simple statement, "I want you to lose weight," without a thorough explanation of the doctor's health plan for weight loss.

2.   Ask any and all necessary questions. If your doctor refuses to answer your inquiries, change doctors.

3.   Physicians should never impose their values on you by criticizing your weight or belittling you.

4.   You have the right to refuse unwanted treatment.

5.   If you fail to lose weight right away (or at all), the doctor should continue to offer help. Unsuccessful patients deserve concern and interest as much as successful ones.

6.   No derogatory language about your size should ever be used by the doctor's staff. Threats, of course, are absolutely not permitted.

7.   You should not have to wait in a doctor's waiting room beyond a reasonable time and certainly not every visit. If you do have consistently long waits, you can suspect the doctor puts patient volume ahead of individual care. Change doctors.

8.   If the doctor gives you pills, you should know what you are taking them for and what possible side effects to expect.

9.   You should receive a good physical examination before any course of treatment is decided. The physical should not take less than twenty minutes, excluding the written history.

10.   The doctor should tell you that you are free to call if you have a problem before your next scheduled visit.

11.   You have the right to expect individual, attentive service from your doctor. If you feel as if you are in a take-a-number medical supermarket, you're in the wrong place. Change doctors.

Bariatricians: the New Diet Doctors

The terms "diet doctor" or "fat doctor" are almost synonymous with "quack" in today's world. They call to mind rainbow pill pushers who cared little for reducing the individual but a great deal for reducing the contents of his or her wallet. Overweight people, people like you and me, even died while under their doubtful care. With such a miserable history, you'd think the best thing overweights could do would be to stay as far from "diet doctors" as possible. Right? Not quite. Do stay away from fly-by-night store front "weight clinics" and doctors who run offices that look like market places for all manner of products and gimmicks. On the other hand, you owe it to yourself to investigate the new diet doctors, who call themselves bariatricians, especially the ones who belong to the American Society of Bariatric Physicians. These men and women actively seek to upgrade the care of overweight patients. Their official journal *Obesity and Bariatric Medicine* is filled with research and caring articles about the problems of dieters. I attended one of their annual conventions, and I was impressed with their efforts to professionalize the treatment of weight problems and set standards for diet doctors. Interestingly enough, a significant number of these physicians have once been overweight themselves, and so were able to "straddle the fence" in understanding their patients. This is not to say that you should drop your own physician if you are getting help and good treatment, but you should be aware that there is a group of 700 physicians across the country who have a *special* interest in you and your problem.

Eating behavior and disorders are complex problems requiring specialized knowledge not every physician has or even wants to acquire. You have a natural right to consult a specialist for your problem of overweight. You can determine if one is in your area by writing The American Society of Bariatric Physicians, 5200 South Quebec, Englewood, Colorado 80111 or telephoning (303) 779-4833.

Your holistic health plan, the personal plan that will bring your body, mind and spirit into harmony at last, will benefit from all the special help and care you can get. A physician is an important resource in your efforts to improve your life. You deserve the best. Go out and get the best.

Choosing the Right Help for Your Mind and Emotions

Nobody needs to tell you that emotional suffering is far too often the by-product of fat. We know, without being told (although we are told), that others think we have some inherent psychological weakness which results in gluttony. We feel more or less consistently insecure in a world which glorifies thinness for its own sake, and this insecurity is likely to produce compensatory overeating. Fat can be painful, so painful that some of us need extra help, psychiatric help to be exact. For two periods in my life, I got extra help for the emotional problems connected with being more than 100 pounds overweight. I didn't lose weight because of psychiatric counseling, but I did gain a better understanding of some of the emotional reasons for my overeating which helped me to apply better self-controls. Most of all, I got supportive feedback which gradually helped me to see myself more realistically and less self-critically as a human being, with the accent on *human.*

Quite often, when an overweight person takes psychotherapy in some form, the therapist won't even concentrate on the weight problem but focuses, instead, on an analysis that will bring about self-acceptance in all areas of the person's life.

Here's how one psychoanalyst, Dr. Douglas H. Ingram of the famous Karen Horney Institute, views the process in *The American Journal of Psychoanalysis:*

Psychoanalytic treatment of fat persons does not differ in its essentials from the psychoanalysis of others. The goal of psychoanalysis, no matter what the presenting complaint, is to help the patient to live more fully and successfully. By stripping away compulsive attitudes and associated behavior through compassionate exploration of unconscious forces, the person emerges with progressive authenticity. As emotional health increases, the person gradually develops the capacity to sustain the process of self-discovery on his own and evolves continuously into a world of deepening subtlety, richness, and meaning. A major function of the psychoanalyst is to redirect attention and involvement that is too sharply focused on excessive fatness and overeating, in order that the person may become better acquainted with his other personal attributes and inner constructive forces . . . The analyst may offer a clear statement of (his intent) for example, "A lot of (your) attention has been taken up by fatness. Without putting that aside entirely, I would also like us to explore other things about you."

Dr. Ingram warns his fellow psychiatrists to know themselves before undertaking work with obese persons. "I am referring to derogatory prejudices about overweight," he says, "in this, the analyst may be heir to dominant cultural biases which he may seek to repress . . ."

The same assertive rights you exercised with the doctor who helps your body are appropriate for the doctor who helps your mind and emotions. You deserve unprejudiced, concerned, competent care. Nothing less will do for you.

Do You Need "Shrinking"?

Not all overweight people need help from the art of psychology to achieve a state of wellness. But some overeaters manifest excessive eating habits which may be helped, or stopped altogether, by effective therapy.

Dr. Floyd K. Garetz, professor of psychiatry at the University of Minnesota, has isolated five reasons why some of us overeat because of our emotions.

1. Some people have food preferences that lead to overweight. These include sugarholics and other obvious starchy-food eaters who simply take in far too many calories.

2. Fast eaters also ingest too much food in a short amount of time.

3. The constant eaters are those who nibble, chew or drink all day in a kind of continuous oral orgy.

4. About ten percent of all overweights are night eaters, taking in the bulk of their calories after all energy expending activities have stopped for the day.

5. Other overweights, about twenty percent of all fat people, are binge eaters. They eat normally most of the time, but can be triggered by anxiety into an enormous food binge.

If one of these problems, or more than one since they can appear in combination, is yours, you may want to get specialized help if you are unable to gain self-control in other ways. The important question you have to ask yourself is whether or not your eating behavior is seriously interfering with your life. Do you turn to food during periods when you are anxious, depressed, bored or under severe stress? If so, therapy is something you may want to consider.

Which therapy is right for you? During the last two decades there has been a proliferation of psychological techniques, so the wise consumer of emotional help has the opportunity to go shopping for the kind of therapy he or she would like best.

Here are brief explanations of some mind therapies you may find helpful.

Adlerian Analysis: Alfred Adler, a disciple of Freud who broke away to form his own goal-oriented therapy did not follow Freud's belief that overeating was related to the sexual drive. Adlerian analysts won't have you searching for penis envy or Oedipal complexes, but will help you discover your self-worth.

Behavior Modification: Treatment of obesity based on the behavioral principles of B.F. Skinner is the most popular of all psychological aids to weight reduction. It is based on four theories:

1. Obesity is a learning disorder.

2. The obese individual is an overeater.

3. There are critical differences in the eating style of obese and nonobese individuals.

4. Training the obese person to eat like a nonobese person will result in weight loss.

A torrent of magazine articles and books, the most authoritative by Dr. Richard B. Stuart, has flooded the diet-starved market in the past decade. The techniques are used by therapy groups, individual dieters, Weight Watchers and Diet Workshops to name but a few. (More information on these groups is contained in Chapter Ten.)

Directed Encounter Groups: An overweight encounter group, led by a sympathetic and unprejudiced professional, provides a setting for the expression of verbal and nonverbal feelings and an exchange of information. An attempt is made to reduce culturally conditioned responses so that participants can operate at a basic emotional level.

est (Erhard Seminar Training): Short-term (two weekends) intensive therapy which seeks to rid an individual of intellectualism and emphasize feelings. Est sessions are held all over the country and seem to attract a variety of young and old, unfamous and celebrity, with a mixed press resulting. Some persons claim to have become much more aware of their feelings; others say what benefits they received were short-term. You may want to read Adelaide Bry's *EST: 60 Hours That Transform Your Life* before you spend the hefty fee.

Gestalt Therapy: This technique, developed by Fritz Perls, emphasizes that incompleteness of personality keeps the individual from fully connecting with his or her environment. Full awareness and an ability to live spontaneously in the present is the goal in this therapy.

118

Group Therapy: Consciousness raising sessions for the over-weight can be especially helpful in getting out feelings of anger, depression and self-contempt and finding that these are not feelings you have because you're bad, but feelings you have because you are fat in a thin chauvinistic world. The general goal of all group therapies is to change attitudes and to help the individual understand that his or her problems are common ones. Reconciliation with the self is the goal. Many diet groups, Overeaters Anonymous in particular, fulfill this function in a nonprofessional way for dieters.

Hypnotherapy: Once widely publicized in the nineteenth century, then largely abandoned, hypnosis has again become a popular method for achieving "painless" weight loss. Defenders of the hypnotic faith claim that they are able to recondition sensory reactions to the stimuli of food so that the mind will not react with hunger. Detractors of the technique say that hypnosis is no more than a super placebo. In other words, patients don't feel hunger because they have been told that they won't feel hunger. According to some specialists, adult overweight women are particularly difficult to hypnotize because of their emotional need to remain in complete control of every situation.

Jungian Analysis: Great emphasis is placed on dream interpretation and on free association, with the idea that it will lead to harmony within the psyche. Like traditional Freudian psychoanalysis, this technique is lengthy and costly.

Primal Therapy: We have all accumulated a pool of pain since childhood, preaches this therapy, which says we must confront it and scream it out (the famous primal scream) in order to effect healing.

Transactional Analysis: This therapy, popularized in the book *I'm O.K., You're O.K.*, states that each person possesses the behavior of a parent, child and adult. The ultimate aim is to help the patient behave in an adult manner most of the time.

Transcendental Meditation (TM): One of the most popular forms of reducing stress (and ultimately your body) in this country today. Using a symbol (mantra) taken from eastern holy books, steady breathing and a comfortable position, the TM practitioner "transcends" consciousness and experiences another awareness. Instructors for this technique can be found all over the country.

You may want to investigate some of these mind-diet techniques, just as you are investigating new body-diet methods. It is part of your holistic search for a lifestyle with which you can live, *really live.*

Experts differ about what constitutes the "obese personality" or, indeed, if there really is one. There does seem to be some consensus that we tend to be passive-aggressive personality types, who rationalize and manipulate in order to resist losing weight. When you add this behavior to the enormous and very conscious mind-body desire that most of us have to move toward health, you can see the stage is set for mental and emotional conflict. If you need objective help in resolving this conflict, by all means, go get it.

The Doctor in Your Holistic Lifestyle

Each of us has a healer inside, a center that strives for physical, emotional and spiritual harmony, both within the "self" and with the rest of the world. It certainly would be foolish to ignore this sense of who you are as a person, but it would be equally foolish to ignore the warnings from your body that tell you you might need a doctor. We overweights are prey to too many diseases, including diabetes, cardiovascular problems, joint and back problems, and chemical imbalances, among others, to reject good medical advice.

The message to you in this chapter is the same message that runs like a strong chain through this book:

1. You are not to blame for your weight problem, but you are taking responsibility for your health today in the best way you can.

2. You will never hang your head in shame.

3. You have the right to good medical care, but you will not take abuse — from anyone — not even a doctor. You will give him or her your money, and if earned, your respect, but you will never give up your own self-esteem.

Part of your lifestyle assault on obesity is self-awareness. Without awareness, you cannot change, and change is what you must have to leave the body-numbing food binges and mind-distorting emotional binges behind.

Become aware, without self-blame, of what you do, how you think and how you act. By assuming control (or mastery) over the directions of your life, you can begin to choose alternative routes, roads that will lead you away from obesity.

You can get help from doctors of the body and the mind, whenever you choose that help, but you can't find anybody else to get rid of your weight problem *for you* and provide you with instant happiness. In the end, you will provide your own happiness, because happiness is up to you. Happiness is a *communication* from the whole you to your conscious self that you are making those basic changes you want to make, that you are using the deep levels of power within yourself. At some level, at this moment, you are responding to the words you are reading. You are examining the pain, hurt, anger and guilt of the past and making an intelligent decision to work for your whole body's health and to create more emotional joy in your own life than you have ever known. After what you've been through, nobody deserves the good life more than you do.

In the next chapter you'll learn that, when it comes to dieting even your best friend or your family can try to do you in. But, as usual, you're one-up on the situation with coping techniques and insights.

HOLISTIC LIFESTYLE CHANGE 8

During the coming week, program yourself to accomplish these goals:

1. Examine your own doctor-patient relationship in light of what you have just read.

2. Make a decision to improve it if you have not already found your own *Dr. Right.*

3. Examine, as best you can, your own emotional health.

4. Make a decision to improve it if you feel you are depressed, indecisive or lacking in self-esteem to the point it interferes with the holistic plan you have for your life.

5. Make a permanent mental note that in any doctor-patient partnership you are the controlling partner and the doctor provides services. The office visit is a learning, as well as healing, experience for you since *you* are your own body manager.

6. Improve your knowledge of holistic healing, perhaps by reading *The Holistic Health Handbook* by the Berkley Holistic Health Center, or other comparable material.

Chapter Nine

Coping With Diet Saboteurs

Everybody knows, especially you, that in the past there has been a high diet failure rate. Surveys indicate that many who lose weight gain it back in a year or two. Much of the problem is, I believe, an overwhelming emphasis on diet or body to the exclusion of the mind and spirit. Holistic dieting, which integrates mind, body and spirit, will make positive inroads on such dismal diet statistics in years to come, just as, happily, holism has made a difference in your life already. Increased consciousness and rejection of "fat guilt" will also turn diet results from negative to positive. But there is another unsolved problem, a little known phenomenon of losing weight so mysterious as to deserve an entire chapter in this book. That phenonenon is diet sabotage. Learning to cope with unexpected reactions to our new thin selves by our circle of relationships will help change future diet statistics in our favor at last.

This diet sabotage business doesn't make sense, does it? How can the ones we love and who love us in return conspire to make us fat again? The answer is they don't — at least most don't do it consciously. When your husband (or wife) comes home with your favorite candy after you've just lost fifty pounds, he's not saying, "Eat it, I want you to be fat again." He's really saying, "I want you to be the person you were, so that I won't have to make so many adjustments in my life."

There are ways of dealing with diet saboteurs. If you have ever had this problem, have it now, or think you will when you reach your natural weight, read on.

First, Get Comfortable with Yourself

When it comes to ease with oneself and self-knowledge, even the thinnest former overweights have a period of adjustment. In order to deal firmly with the changes others have to make in their lives, it's a good idea to deal with our own comfortability first. How do you feel about being thin?

Sometimes we don't feel thin at all; we can even feel like strangers to ourselves. Some of us, at least for a period of time, can totally reject our new bodies. "It's not me," we say, "it's some-one else." The more weight we lose, the more apt we are to feel such disorientation. Here are some ways we can become more comfortable with our new selves:

1. *Believe what you see.* When you look in the mirror and your thighs don't touch, your arms hang at your sides instead of at a fat-induced forty-five degree angle and you count only one chin, then you *are* thin.

2. *Be sensitive, but not over-sensitive.* Don't think others are ex-pecting too much of you now that you're thin. Chances are others are more tolerant of you than you are of yourself.

3. *Don't make excessive demands on yourself.* You can't make up for lost "fat years" in a day. Take on new activities one at a time, so that you don't overload and short-cut the delicate new coping circuits you are slowly developing.

4. *Build your self-esteem.* You have already greatly improved your positive feeling for yourself through the process of losing weight. Now start acting like a self-loving, confident person. Don't explain yourself and your actions too much. Try not to say, "I'm sorry," overmuch or for imagined faults. Apologetic behavior (that's the way you acted because you felt guilty and fat) is simply unnecessary at any size.

5. *Face fear.* One of the most pervasive of all feelings is fear. If you are afraid that you won't measure up to other thin people, or worse yet, that you'll get fat again, then you are concentrating on a very negative feeling. Take a few minutes at the beginning of each day to view the world as a good place instead of dangerous and uncertain. (You might try a morale-boosting reading ex-perience. I can, immodestly, recommend my book *The Thin Book* which will give you daily reinforcement.)

Each new day will provide stimulating experiences which come only *because* your new life is uncertain. You are no longer "con-trolling" your feelings and your environment with extra food, so that life *will* bring surprises. Don't be afraid of them; they are part of your aliveness.

Now that you are beginning to feel less dis-ease with your new, slim body and your new holistic thinking systems as well, you may notice that others in your circle of relationships are acting strangely. The closer they are, (husband, wife, children, parents) the more intense their reaction, and it can be negative. What!

How can this be? After you've gone to all the trouble (yes, and suffered, too) to lose weight, the least they could do is praise your marvelous achievement. Right? Not necessarily. Now, when you are at the pinnacle of your success, may be just the time that they balk and begin to do and say things which, for all the world, look like sabotage, like they actually wanted you to be fat again. How could they be so cruel? No others in your life know better than they how miserable being fat made you. Why aren't they as happy as you are? Why are they doing and saying such terrible things? Why, indeed?

The "Fat Family" System

"Families are really intricate systems," says Dr. Trudy Helmlinger, a Sacramento, California family and marriage counselor. "When one person changes within the system it affects all the other members usually in a negative way by creating anxiety."

Psychologist Helmlinger goes on to say that this anxiety can manifest itself in two ways: the anxious family member either withdraws or acts out anger. "Either way," Dr. Helmlinger adds, "the first thing they try to do is change a person back."

Let's say, for illustration, that a family has an overweight mother. Everybody in that family system has adjusted his or her behavior to the fact that mom is fat. They are *dependent* on her fatness. For example, because mother is fat, in our imaginary family, the children can expect lots of baked goodies when they come home from school and a parent who is more than eager to chauffeur them around to make up for her "fat shortcomings." The husband can expect a submissive wife who defers to his opinions, one who spends very little money on her wardrobe and who allows him to nag her at meals and feel a little bit superior.

What happens? Mom goes on a diet, loses fifty pounds and changes her way of thinking about herself. She doesn't have as much time to bake or chauffeur, since she is out shopping for attractive new clothes, attending interesting classes or maybe getting a new job. No one can feel superior or nag her at meals because she is a more disciplined eater than any other family member. The result? The family system is topsy-turvy. Everybody is anxious because they *counted* on mom to always stay the way she was.

"Suddenly," says Dr. Helmlinger, explaining how the family feels, "it's almost like they don't know what to do with their hands!"

What a dilemma! As you lose weight and become more self-actualizing, you are going to need their approval, but at the same time, you are becoming less dependent on them and they must become less dependent on you.

WARNING. At this point, the adjustments can prove to be all too much to bear. You can begin to feel guilty and gain the weight back to avoid any further family disruption.

You and your family can experience all this trauma without ever knowing what you are feeling or why.

Although it would be false to say that diet sabotage is a "woman's problem," because it happens to men and even children, in truth it happens to women more often because more women are overweight and more women go on diets to lose weight. Nevertheless, regardless of your sex or age, does any part of the preceding scenario sound familiar? If it does, here's what you can do about it, and in so doing, reduce your chances of regaining your hard-won weight loss.

Sidestepping Sabotage

I have been amazed (and concerned) to read in "advice to the overweight" columns and books that the way to combat diet sabotage is to ignore it, fight it, or try to help the saboteurs to see the error of their ways. These methods will have exactly the opposite effect from what is intended, actually *increasing* resistance to our change. None of these methods will work because *there is nothing in it for the saboteur.*

In the first place, most of them are well-meaning and unaware that they resent our change, even unaware that our changing has forced adjustments in their own relationships with us. The very last thing we want to do is to add to their burden by showing them their mistakes, if we want their cooperation. And cooperation is precisely what we do want. Here's how we can get it.

Early in your holistic lifestyle assault on your own weight problem, sit down with your family and COMMUNICATE. (You won't want to tell them they are going to try and sabotage your weight loss, because they would be very hurt and angry at the very idea. That's just an insight which you will have to share with your overweight friends, but *not* with your family.) Communicate your idea that as you lose weight, the family as a whole may have some adjustments to make. Get out a sheet of paper and make a list of the positive changes and (what they see as) negative changes. If your conversation will be on an intimate level, you may want to have two communication sessions, one with your children and one with your spouse. Initiate the plan-ahead conversation with this question: What kinds of changes do you think the family will undergo if I lose weight? Most of the responses will be unrealistically positive, so that you will have to steer the conversation to the other possibilities mentioned in the scenario about the imaginary family earlier in this chapter. And you will want to add things that are peculiar to your own family. This form of specific communication helps to alert your family to the possibility of change and also tips them off that the changes are tied to your weight loss.

Later, as you lose weight and your family begins to alter the way they relate to you, *you are going to have to give them rewards*. Remember, when you're losing weight you get more or less continuous rewards because you feel better and look better. You are making adjustments in your life and getting rewards. But your family is making adjustments in their lives and *not* getting rewards. There's nothing mysterious about giving rewards. Simply remember to take time out to say, "You're more important to me now than you have ever been," or "I appreciate some of the things you're going through because of my change." This kind of recognition coupled with the initial communication you have had can make a big difference if you remember to continue to give them "strokes" for their acceptance of the new you.

Sure, it may be a bit of extra trouble, but it will be worth it if you lessen or do away with diet sabotage. And think of it this way. Knowing in advance how the family system for overweights works can give you more control over what happens to you in your life, a far better control than overeating, a substitute control that is very low-calorie.

What Your Family Can Do For You; What You Can Do For Your Family

Don't misunderstand what has been said. None of the above should be construed to mean that families shouldn't support their dieting members. They can and they should.

1. Your family should not NAG. Who needs to tell us we're fat?

2. Your family should not buy you boobytrap gifts. Who needs chocolate bonbons? Gifts should be personal — and nonedible.

3. Your family should try to eat foods the dieting member eats. Most diets are more nutritious than regular family fare anyway,

so family members can get their goodies on the side or away from home if they must have them.

4. Your family should remember that meal schedules may be tighter. The dieting member may have to eat early if the family is late.

It is true that your family has an obligation to help you in every way they can. After all, that's why human beings invented the family unit. But you also have an obligation to your family.

1. You should give praise for praise. It's wonderful when your husband, wife or children say, "I know you're trying hard. Keep it up." But don't forget to respond, "I really appreciate your wonderful support ."

2. You should give your family "ego food." Let them know, spontaneously, how valuable they are to you and that you haven't gotten a "swelled head" from a thin body.

3. You should be understanding of your family. Don't complain that, after all the trouble you went to to get a new figure "for them," they don't appreciate you enough. They have problems accepting the new you, as you well know, so expect that they may not always be in the mood to praise your really wonderful accomplishment. Wait. They will feel better about things in a short while, especially if you continue to reinforce their positive efforts.

Friends, Co-workers and Everyone Else

According to surveys, about 63 percent of our help (or sabotage) while dieting will come from our families, leaving 37 percent to come from all other relationships. That's natural. The closer the relationship, the more intense it is and the more helpful or hurtful it can be. The more distant the relationship — those outside our families — the less involvement they can have with our weight loss and the less they will have to adjust their own lives.

It's only fair to tell you, though, that everyone in our lives will react to our change to some degree. They will react not only to psychological changes but also to our physical change. Dr. Jerome D. Oreland at San Francisco Children's Hospital and Adult Medical Center believes that physical change is basically related to a person's sense of self-continuity and is threatening to observe. One woman patient of his reported that even her customers and employees tried to interfere with her weight loss because of this perceived threat.

After family, friends are most likely to react strangely once you start to pare down your familiar fat shape. They just don't like to see radical changes in those around them, so they say irrational things like, "You're losing too much weight. I liked you better when you were heavier," or "Aren't you worried about being too flabby?"

Now, chances are you aren't losing too much weight. Ten to one, you're not even halfway to your goal. If that's true, you can suspect the old sabotage game, and apply the same solution as you did for your familiy. For really close friends, you may want to sit down and talk to them about how your weight loss may bring a physical change but won't make any difference in your friendship. You may want to give them praise for their support and, in other ways, reassure them that *their* adjustments haven't gone unnoticed or unappreciated. The important thing with friends, co-workers and, indeed, all your relationships is that you give them the same rewards for adjusting to your change as you expect from them for losing weight. Relationships are a two-way street whether you are overweight, thin or still losing.

Don't Forget to Be Assertive

If you are having serious trouble with diet saboteurs in or out of your family, it may also be helpful for you to reread Chapters Four and Five on assertiveness for the overweight. Sabotage, after all, is an unconscious effort to manipulate you into doing what makes others feel more comfortable.

One caution seems appropriate here, especially when you are dealing with your family or close friends. How many times have you recapped an argument in your mind and decided that the other person must have been at fault since your words were sweet and reasonable. Your memory may be right as far as it goes, but you've omitted the all-important tone of voice and body gestures that went with your words. If they were negative or aggressive, your sweet words will be seen by others as insincere or sarcastic.

You have the right to be thin and to live your life in your own interest, unmanipulated by others, even your own family or best friends. As you have read time and again in these pages, you are capable of honest confrontation because you value and respect yourself and expect others to value and respect you, too. Such an attitude melts the bars of your fat cell faster than the blow torch of resentment or aggression.

It doesn't happen often, but what if you've tried everything to cope with a diet saboteur? You've communicated that there will be a change when you're thin, given praise for praise and continued to give strokes during your period of weight loss and after. You've done everything by the book, but the saboteur is just too threatened by the new, thin you. If there is nothing more you can do, you must ask yourself the question: how important is this relationship to me? It's a tough question, but you've had tough ones before. In the end, all your relationships must adjust to your new body, mind and spirit or you must adjust to their concept of you. It is as simple as that. Which life will you live? Yours? Or theirs?

"We do our best when the center of our lives is lodged in our own substance rather than in the hands of other people," writes Dr. Theodore Rubin in his book *Alive and Fat and Thinning in America*. Amen to that.

Ten Sabotage Boobytraps and How to Disarm Them

1. **The Food Trap:** Your wife serves tempting dishes (or your husband brings home your binge foods) when she knows you are serious about losing weight. Honestly, what's so strange about that? Most of us overweights have reacted with pleasure to certain foods until we have conditioned those around us to express love in that way. (If you've been married ten years, you've eaten more than 11,000 meals together.) Begin to show your affection for your wife (or husband) in a variety of other ways so that food will no longer be a symbol of love in your relationship.

2. **The People Pleaser Trap:** One of the most effective ways you can be blown right off your diet is to have gone on one for the wrong reasons. If you're trying to lose weight to please someone else, the first time they make you angry you're going to do the best get-even thing you can think of. That's right. EAT! The solution is to go on a diet or make any change in your way of living because *you* want to do it for your own sake. We overweights do best when *we* are in charge of our lives.

3. **The "Superior-to-thou" Trap:** It pains me to say that some of us successful dieters go through a period when we think a bit too highly of our accomplishments. If we can lose weight, we sweetly reason, then our spouses ought to be able to quit smoking, our children make straight-A averages and our friends give up their bad habits, too. This can cause any support we get from them to melt away, and they may want to sabotage us "up to size" again. It

130

is certainly true that we have done a difficult and wonderful thing for ourselves, but it is not true that we have answers for everybody. If our integrated holistic lifestyle is positively changing our lives, we will not be able to keep people from asking us what we're doing. Attraction, rather than detraction is the answer.

4. **The Martyr Trap:** An extension of the "superior-to-thou" trap is when we begin to feel unfairly picked-on. We throw the great question heavenward: "Why me?" We feel an overwhelming sense of responsibility for our weight problem, while people all around us seem to zip through life with a minimum of troubles. We ask, "Why do they get to eat what they want while I have to diet?"

You may be right. You may have been dealt a bad genetic hand. So what! You've still got the same choices you always had. You can insist on diet martyrdom, but you should know the path to the refrigerator is drenched in "poor me" tears. It is up to you. It always is.

5. **The Watch Dog Trap:** You are going on vacation or to a party and you insist that your spouse or friend guard you from self-inflicted food. "Now, promise you'll watch me and don't let me have any sweets," you plead. Extracting such a promise does two unfair things. It places the burden of your conscience onto another, and it is a subtle message to your own brain that you aren't really in control of what you eat. If you aren't in control, you're in trouble. Don't use others as tools; they can support you but they can't live for you.

6. **The Nostalgia Trap:** Mates of both sexes who have low ego problems themselves are afraid that as we grow thinner, they are not going to be able to compete for our affections. Your mate might say, "I loved you just as much when you were heavy," or worse yet, "I don't like you this way." Don't allow yourself to be appealed to on the basis that yesterday's fat old you was a better mate and that the way to make your spouse happy is to get fat all over again. Encourage mates to think well of themselves. Show you find them attractive and desirable no matter what size you are.

7. **The Pleasure Trap:** One of the cardinal precepts of diet dining is to always eat in pleasant company. One diet wit responded to that advice with: "Does this mean I can't eat with my family?" No, but it does mean that it is more important than ever, for everybody's sake, to assure that mealtimes are as pleasant as possible. We overweights are oral people. We enjoy the act of

eating for its own sake. To have this pleasure disturbed by others is to create stress at a vulnerable point. Keep potential arguments for another time — any other time — but mealtime.

8. **The Security Trap:** When you are overweight, you can usually be counted on to stay in one place. If you are married, you're always at home, always ready to do things that show others (while you may be fat) that you are certainly devoted. Thin people don't mean to exploit our guilt, but they can grow to expect the personal service it generates. When we lose our extra pounds, become more socially active and spend more time on ourselves, those around us can feel less secure. In time, you can help mates understand that the more active, thinner you are is not a rejection of them, but an affirmation of yourself. You certainly won't make your marriage more secure by regaining lost weight.

9. **The Sex Trap:** Some predatory males (and liberated females) look upon the newly fat-free in the same way that they view the divorced or widowed — as sex-starved. True, overweights often have a voluptuous personality that can be misinterpreted as promiscuous. Watch out for sex vultures. Nobody likes to be exploited for his or her body, even if they are newly proud of it.

10. **The Criticism Trap:** The biggest boobytrap of all is the amount of (unknowing) sabotaging criticism you will get, especially right after you've lost your weight. As you become more self-assertive, those for whom you have played the victim are going to be upset. They are going to want you to "be your old self again." If you recognize this criticizing behavior, but only reinforce the supportive things they do, the criticism will stop. Remember they aren't thinking of what is best for you, but of what is best for themselves. You must show them by your own behavior that your new lifestyle will bring the entire family closer together, since you are obviously going to be a happier, whole person. In the end, your success is everybody's success.

Yes, the man or woman you love best, the one you have promised to love, honor and cherish, may be trying to sabotage your new body and dearest wish. Don't be too hard on your mate. Remember they wouldn't do it, knowingly or unknowingly, if they didn't love you and want to keep you. Just don't expect too much from them as you emerge from your fat cell, and they'll soon adjust, especially if you give them "strokes" for adjusting. It might be well to remember also, that part of your diet success, according to a *Journal of the American Dietetic Association* study, you owe to the simple fact that you *are* married. Researchers discovered that marriage was one of the solid predictors of weight-loss success.

How to Be a Charming Guest Without Overeating

Now that you're thinner, more integrated, you may find yourself sought-after socially. Family and friends may even want to show you off a bit. Of course, these occasions in your honor couldn't turn into a gastronomical debauch, could they? Couldn't they?

At one party given for me after I'd lost 100 pounds, the sweetly sabotaging hostess assured me it was perfectly all right to eat a piece of her famous cheesecake. "After all," she said, "I only bake it once a year. You couldn't get fat on *that*."

What, besides becoming anti-social, can we overweights (just thin or still losing) do? First, we can avoid all social functions whose only excuse for happening is food and drink; for example, progressive dinners, pizza and beer or wine and cheese parties.

Second, and most important, we can meet a host's insistence with a larger helping of polite resistance. "No, thank you, I *never* eat that at *any* time."

Next, you can try resisting with humor, if that's your style. "Thank you, no. If I eat that tonight, my skin won't fit tomorrow."

Or be a snob. "Oh, my *dear*, I never eat oysters in that rich sauce. We cruised to Europe last summer, you know, and oysters *au naturel* were the rage at all the best restaurants."

Try sneakery, if the host has a reputation for keeping the drinks coming. Bring a diet 7-Up in your purse and surreptitiously fill your glass, also chock-full of ice cubes, with this no-cal "martini."

When all else fails — LIE. "My doctor has ordered me not to eat (or drink) that. Liver disease, you know." Hold your right side as you say this and grimace with pain. It helps the tale if you can wear a slightly yellowed expression.

No one can force you to eat anything you don't really want to eat. I have been urged, prodded and coerced by the best of them, but I have yet to experience force-feeding.

Don't be overly concerned about having to become a hermit just as you are coming out of your fat cell. Most hosts today inquire if you have food preferences or problems; or, if they don't inquire, most of them know that weight-consciousness is the norm and provide a simple entree.

If you are having trouble controlling your eating at parties, try these two steps:

Step one. Give yourself a positive talk before you go. Tell yourself that you *can* manage your eating and drinking at parties, and that you will concentrate on enjoying your friends. Your satisfaction will come from social contact, not hors d'oeuvres.

Step two. Tell yourself that *nobody is looking at your plate.* So many times because we are very self-aware, we think others are overly interested in everything we do. Actually others are concerned about themselves. If you have always been so self-conscious that you doubt this, try this little experiment. Take a group picture the next time you are at a party, using one of the instant cameras. Pass the picture around without telling anyone about your little experiment. Who do people look at in the picture first? Themselves. Now, look at the picture yourself. Who do you look at first? Yourself. Do you get the picture?

Eat and drink what you have to eat and drink for your body, mind and spirit health program. You are the one who will be looking at you — for the rest of your life.

Holistic Coping

The German philosopher Goethe gave us a unique definition of self-awareness. The real meaning of self-knowledge, he said, lies in taking notice of oneself in relation to other people and to the world.

This is especially true for us overweights when we deal with potential diet saboteurs. For so long we have been advised to be defensive, to expect, yes even demand, attention in the form of continuous support from others. As you can see from this chapter, that is a totally unrealistic, psychologically impractical expectation on our part. Quite without knowing it, most everybody acts in their own self-interest. To constantly expect others to give praise when their own lives are being negatively affected is to expect them to behave like saints. How many of us are married to saints? Isn't it more realistic, and downright practical, to take on ourselves some of the responsibility for our family or friend's adjustment to our new image? Of course, we can't be totally responsible, but we can recognize that they are having a difficult time and try in the ways outlined in this chapter to make it a little easier for them. Not only will you capture the heart of any unknowing saboteur, but by showing this kind of strength you enhance your own self-esteem. Isn't it interesting how our positive actions always come back to us?

Coping holistically with diet sabotage is a good example of what health expert Leonard Duhl calls "synchronicity." The goal of holistic health quite simply extends from our relationship with self to others, and to the environment. Whatever you want to call it — harmony, balance, synchronicity — the clear message is that our personal concept of wholeness must extend beyond self-integration to integration with our universe.

Now that you are more open to the effect your weight loss and personality change have on others, try to open yourself to the positive effect others, in particular other overweights, can have on you. In the next chapter, we'll explore another aspect of your life-style assault on obesity — the world of diet clubs. Your questions will be answered: Do you need their help? Which one is right for you? Where are they and what will they cost? In short, a thorough handbook on the growing diet group scene.

HOLISTIC LIFESTYLE CHANGE 9

Remember that reading without doing is like eating without swallowing, and make the following changes in your life.

1. If you have had, now have or expect to have problems with diet saboteurs, sit down right now and make a plan of action based on the principles in this chapter and your own situation.

2. Accept the idea completely that you, not anybody else, are responsible for your health.

3. Reread the ten sabotage boobytraps. How many of them have you fallen into? How will you arm yourself against these traps in the future?

4. Commit yourself to the idea that every social event or holiday will not be turned into an oral orgy no matter how much pressure you get from the host or hostess.

5. Believe in your right to thinness, but help those around you who have trouble with it in every way you can, but one. You don't owe them getting fat again. No healthy relationship demands it. No unhealthy relationship deserves it.

Chapter Ten

How Diet Clubs Can Help You

Fifteen years ago, I attended my first diet group meeting. I didn't know what to expect; indeed, I didn't really *want* to be there, but I was desperate for help. During that beautiful hour and a half, I heard other overweights, rational and intelligent people, talk about the problems fat had caused in their lives and how they have overcome them. I was so overwhelmed by a feeling of being "at home" that to my embarrassment, I began to cry. A loving woman near me reached for my hand and said quietly, "I know what you are feeling," and I immediately understood that she did. Although I have been to hundreds of diet group meetings all over the United States in the years since, that first one remains in my mind as the epitome of what the right diet group can do for an unhappy overweight.

All diet groups are not alike. Most of the major national and international organizations are quite different, each with a "personality" of its own. The trick for every overweight who wants maximum help is to match his or her personality to the right group. This chapter will help you do that for yourself. But first, let's look at the self-help diet group picture, a modern phenomenon.

The Diet Tribes

Our ancestors, who banded together to survive, eating only an occasional mastodon steak medium-rare, or wild berries from the bush and natural roots from the fields, would have thought our world of food plenty an earthly paradise. Yet, this very plenty has forced many of early man's sons and daughters to band together once again, not to share food this time, but to survive its abundance. These modern-day tribes we call diet groups are today's answer to the age-old problem of sustaining life. Our forefathers needed the strength of a tribe to get more food to eat; their descendents need the strength of numbers to stop overeating.

What are diet groups about and how do they work? You should know a bit of their dynamics before you consider joining. The approach of most self-help groups is really quite old-fashioned. They provide support and encouragement, give rewards for success, stress such ancient values as compassion and reliance on a higher power and give each other cheery, can-do tips on how to deal with dieting. Most groups have a definite esprit de corps, which helps overweight people rejected by thin chauvinistic society feel accepted at last.

Frankly, many fat people are attracted to diet groups for a practical reason — they work. One recent study at Brown University's Butler Hospital found that people who dieted in a group lost nearly 10 pounds in ten weeks as opposed to four pounds lost by people on the same diet but whose only contact was by mail. *People* made the difference.

"Fat people are usually givers and takers," says Dr. Theodore Rubin, "they are 'people people,' or in other words, they *need* people, especially during difficult times."

Just how do self-help groups work? What do they do for you? Another study, again from Brown University, solves the mystery. The psychologists at Brown used a variety of self-help groups, including TOPS (Take Off Pounds Sensibly) and Overeaters Anonymous, and found diet groups did four things for overweights:

1. *The groups provided social involvement or fellowship.* Significantly, this social aspect of diet groups was rated more important by the participants of this study than its diet help, which only strengthens Dr. Rubin's contention that overweights, like the song says, are "people who need people."

2. *The groups helped members in reaching goals.* Instead of floating helplessly in a sea of fat-forming food, diet group members are set on a well-charted course to thinness.

3. *The groups helped overweights to understand and accept their problems.* It's difficult, if not impossible, to maintain a "poor baby" attitude if, all around you, others are losing weight.

4. *The groups facilitated members' personal growth.* Success breeds success. when you begin to increase in self-esteem, you can begin to tackle other troublesome living problems.

These same diet-group members when asked specifically *why* their group had been effective for them attributed it to:

1. A supportive, accepting environment.
2. A change in the way they viewed their weight problem.
3. More understanding of themselves and their problems.
4. Learning that it was possible to achieve their goals.

One diet group member I met long ago explained the meaning of self-help groups to me in even more simple terms. "I can place my hands under this side," he said, grasping the edge of a large table, "and I can't lift it alone. But if others get around the table and lift, too, then I can do with their help what I was never able to do alone."

Nevertheless, there are people who should not join diet self-help groups. It may require more involvement than they want and create additional stress, which, Lord knows, no overweight needs. Before you consider joining any self-help group, look over the Diet Group Personality Checklist on page 152 to see if such a move is one you should seriously consider.

If you don't score seven or more on the Checklist questions with a Yes, that doesn't necessarily mean you wouldn't benefit from diet group membership. It does mean that you should be all the more careful in matching your personality with the personality of the diet group.

The "Shall I Join?" Conflict

"Groups meet people's need to belong," says Dr. Trudy Helmlinger of the Eskaton Mental Health Clinic. "But people live in conflict with this need because nobody wants to think they're dependent on others. They're afraid of losing their control and their identity."

But you can resolve this human need in diet groups. Overweights (and other people as well) find a welcome duality in groups, says Dr. Helmlinger. If you are open and like to talk about your problems, groups provide a platform, but if you want to hide in a group, you can do that, too.

If you decide to join a self-help diet group or are already a member, there are many benefits but there are also two potential problems of which you'll want to be aware. The two are:

The Pedestal Pitfall: When you lose a great deal of weight, your entire personality changes. You dress and speak more assertively. You glow with health and vitality. More than a little stardust trails in your wake. What happens? You may find yourself high on the group's pedestal. What then? A strange thing can happen. Members of your group can start to sabotage you. Impossible? Not quite. People, even fat people, have ambivalent feelings about others that they perceive are above them. If they find it hard on their necks to keep looking up at you, they might not mind your falling. It doesn't seem to matter that they put you up there in the first place.

In the meantime, you're having some hard feelings of your own, standing on your marble pedestal. Other group members seem to need too much from you. You feel anger. You feel used.

To avoid the Pedestal Pitfall, you should remember that a marvelous thing has happened to you. You have a whole, natural body again and you're damned grateful. You really want to help others achive what you have, but you insist on your right to privacy and your right to be *one of the group* not someone apart from it, no matter how rarified the apartness. After all, you came into the group so you could finally become an insider.

Keep your sense of balance and humor and you won't have the negative feelings that could eventually lead from pedestal to refrigerator.

Dropout Guilt: Many self-help diet groups suggest in various ways that membership, if it is to be effective, must be permanent. In other words, if you discontinue the group's program you can *expect* to return to overeating and regain all your lost weight. Whether or not this is always true or is ever true is a matter of ideological faith since there is no research on the subject. It is apparent, however, that many diet group members believe this, true or not. What happens if you decide to change diet groups or you think you'd just like to stop altogether? What happens, all too often, is guilt, diet-shattering guilt and, even worse, the prophecy of a return to overeating comes true. The "once an overeater, always an overeater" theory is believed to an almost brainwashing degree, and the belief can *cause* you to make it come true. This would seem to leave overweights with two choices: stay in the group for life, or leave and regain lost weight. Not so. There is another option, if you wish to exercise it, one that will help to wipe out diet group dropout guilt for good.

1. Choose the right time. The time to leave is when more things are going on in your life than your weight.

2. Tell yourself from the very beginning that you retain the right to stay or leave the group as you choose.

3. Use positive terminology if you do decide to leave. You're not dropping out, you're *graduating*.

4. Have a system for leaving which makes the transition positive. If there's a silent (but implied) contract between you and your

group which tells you that you're going to fall on your face if you leave, then you're going to have to get very angry in order to psyche yourself into leaving. You eliminate the need for such anger if you:

   a. Tell yourself that you have the right to try to keep your weight off on your own — to move from dependency to independency.

   b. That you have the right to come back to the group at a later time, if you want to.

   5. Develop a positive plan for saying goodbye. Let the group know in advance (at least three weeks) so that they have a chance to tell you how much they're going to miss you and you'll have a chance to tell them how hard you're going to work. In this way you are leaving in a manner which causes you the least guilt and the group the least anxiety.

You may never decide to leave or change your diet group, if that's where you want to be. The point is not to exchange your fat cell for a group prison.

Yes, there are some group problems which you can learn to handle, but by far, groups are more positive than negative for the majority of overweights.

An interesting and very positive aspect of group participation discovered in a university study points to the ability of diet group members to reach out for other sources of help. People who once had doubts about groups in the first place report that group membership helped them become more open to such alternative sources of aid as religion, friends, other kinds of groups, family and books. They become true seekers, and in a holistic sense, assumed increased responsibility for their own well-being.

Shopping for the Right Group

Diet groups, like Shakespeare's Cleopatra, are of infinite variety. Each of them has a program and personality all its own, which you should try to match to your own personality needs. This may require you to shop around until you find just the right diet group "marriage" for you. Just like any intelligent, conscientious shopper you will want to make comparisons and check off the list of things you expect from a self-help diet group. Here is what you should look for before joining:

   1. Diet groups should be nonthreatening in their helping techniques, never ridiculing or embarrassing. If they're not, LEAVE IMMEDIATELY.

2. Ask how much it costs, not just the basic fees but any extras you may be expected to buy.

3. If the group's philosophy is not explained during the meeting, ask a member or the lecturer. Satisfy yourself that you could adjust emotionally to the group's focus.

4. Check out the recommended diet. Ask where the diet comes from and whether or not it is nutritionally sound, varied and tailored to special conditions, such as adolescence, pregnancy and male-female differences. If the group advocates fasting and has no medical supervision, GET OUT.

5. Determine whether or not the group advocates a total program of diet, exercise and emotional uplift.

6. Look around for success. Notice how many are losing weight and how many members have maintained their weight loss.

On balance, most diet groups, particularly the Big Four (Weight Watchers, Diet Workshop, TOPS and Overeaters Anonymous), are often helpful experiences, especially if you find it difficult to diet alone. Be selective and keep your options open and you should do very well. Check the Diet Group Registry at the end of the chapter for addresses.

Take a Look at the "Big Four" Diet Groups

It is appropriate to start this diet group roundup of top self-help groups with TOPS (for Take Off Pounds Sensibly), since it is the mother of all weight losing organizations. Every succeeding group, and every diet group member, owes a debt of gratitude to TOPS founder Esther S. Manz, who got together with a few overweight housewives in 1948 and started it all.

TOPS: Statistically, TOPS is a nonprofit organization with more than 12,500 groups and more than 338,000 members in every state and 28 foreign countries. During a recent year, members counted a total weight loss of 1,166 tons. That's 2,332,000 pounds! It is financed by nominal membership dues and, unlike the other three national organizations, sends its members to their family doctors for physical checkups and diets.

Of the Big Four, TOPS is the most old-fashioned. Meetings I have attended had the feeling of a good-natured neighborhood coffee klatch. I was instantly made to feel welcome.

TOPS literature specifies private weekly weigh-ins, since your weight is your own business. Due to space limitations in certain meetings, I found the injunction was not always adhered to, although only weight gain or loss were mentioned aloud during meetings.

If you scored Yes on Question 9 in the Diet Group Personality Checklist earlier in this chapter, you will feel particularly comfortable in TOPS. Keen competition over pounds lost is one of the main features of the program. But it doesn't stop there. An elaborate system of recognition and rewards boosts your spirits and helps keep you on the track. Each chapter crowns a queen (men have separate chapters and, naturally, crown kings) based on an individual's weight loss, charm and general personality improvement after weight loss.

Once TOPS members reach their weight goal, they are encouraged to join KOPS (for Keep Off Pounds Sensibly) where the cycle of competition and rewards continues to help them maintain their new figures.

What can you expect at your first meeting? Conviviality is the hallmark of most TOPS groups. With their songbook, which has set nearly every well-known, often-sung tune to new diet lyrics, you may have the feeling that you have walked into a boozeless party. There are even games and skits. But aside from the often manic fun is a genuine atmosphere of warmth and caring for each other which is effortlessly extended to the newcomer.

Although members openly discuss the problems of obesity, the spiritual and emotional side of overeating has been neglected by TOPS until recently. Research with their own members has provided TOPS headquarters with specific material on the psychological aspects of overweight which they are sending to their groups for use as discussion topics.

The organization publishes TOPS NEWS, a cheery, subscription magazine with recipes, pictures of happy losers, diet tips and awards, a perfect illustration of what is probably the most *upbeat* of all the diet groups.

Overeaters Anonymous: Founded in 1960 after a fat, unhappy Los Angeles housewife attended a Gamblers Anonymous meeting, OA today numbers more than 3,700 groups in 16 countries.

Although most diet groups claim kinship with Alcoholics Anonymous, they are no more than poor step-sisters compared with Overeaters Anonymous, which has taken to itself the famous "12 Steps" of AA, changing only the word "alcohol" to the word "food."

Essentially, OA believes that the obese are sufferers of a

disease called compulsive overeating, a disease which will succumb to five life changes:

1. *Abstinence* from compulsive overeating by adherence to OA's dietary program and elimination of individual binge foods.

2. *Sponsorship* of a newcomer by a veteran member who shows the "baby" (new member) how to adopt behavior compatible to losing weight and who serves as a potent model of success.

3. *Telephone calls* between meetings which act as the OA "lifeline" from member to member, providing all-important daily contact with an advocate of the OA lifestyle.

4. *Anonymity* which is the spiritual foundation of OA, so that members may say whatever they please in meetings without fear that it will go beyond the room. In a more obscure way, anonymity is defined as "humility" in that members may not reveal their affiliation on a public level in order that they not become puffed-up with pride, fall down and overeat, thus hurting the reputation of the group.

5. *Literature reading,* which is an integral part of OA's program, is aimed at total reeducation of the "compulsive personality."

Two basic concepts underlie this OA program. One says that a *Power greater and outside* the overeater can control a member's eating problem where he or she may have failed many times. Number two says that an overeater must *surrender* his or her ego to this Higher Power in order to make the program work. This is, admittedly, strong stuff for many overweights but "salvation" for as many others.

OA's meetings, more than any other self-help diet group, have the distinct flavor of the evangelical tent meeting. Individual members are encouraged to stand up and share their experience, strength and hope with other members, the idea being to help others and, by so doing, to shore up their own resolve. Because many members share weekly their stories of misery, struggle and deliverance, some have become brilliant speakers able to move crowds to tears and laughter-filled emotional highs. Such a meeting is the kind of cathartic, spiritual experience every overweight should have at least once, whether they are interested in making OA their own diet group or not.

The atmosphere in OA is more emotionally tense than in TOPS. No songs, skits or weigh-ins lighten the meetings, although there is often relief in the form of genuine humor aimed at individual experiences with fat. While the tone is serious and spiritual, it is not religious. Members are not required to believe in a specific Higher Power, but may choose nature or even the group as a source for power greater than their own.

Did you score Yes on Question 8 in the Diet Group Personality Checklist? If you did, you may like OA very much. Or check the OA test, "Are You a Compulsive Overeater?," on page 151 to see if you may belong with this group; but even if you don't you should treat yourself to a unique experience by attending at least one meeting.

Weight Watchers: The next diet self-help group to appear (in 1963) was Weight Watchers, the brainchild of a Long Island housewife named Jean Nidetch. A year earlier Jean had gone on the New York City Health Department diet and lost 72 pounds, a loss which attracted friends and neighbors to seek her help. Having a natural gift of gab, Jean was soon lecturing at the forerunners of Weight Watcher's classes, and these virtually exploded into an international weight-losing corporation which made her a celebrity and quite possibly a millionaire several times over.

Unlike TOPS and OA which are nonprofit, Weight Watchers is very much for profit, selling a variety of low-calorie products, ready-made frozen "program" meals, books, a monthly magazine plus licensing regional franchise operations and WW camps for overweight adults and youngsters.

But making money doesn't seem to get in the way of Weight Watchers being able to help fat people, since more than eight million people have enrolled in more than 12,000 classes. (There is some question if all those people were first-timers. I, alone, accounted for five of those eight million, joining and dropping and rejoining again more than a decade ago.)

Weight Watchers classes have changed considerably in recent years, so if you haven't tried them for a time, you may want to give them another chance. Nutrition is emphasized and behavioral training has been added to teach WW members self-control. Many foods formerly on the no-no list are now permitted, so that the onerous (to some) fish and liver regimen doesn't look like the same diet at all.

Three basic plans teach overweights to satisfy their appetites with the right foods during weight loss, approaching their goal weight and after goal weight has been achieved. But there is much more to WW meetings than eating plans. The atmosphere is cordial, the cost is not high (compared with other commercial or salon programs) and the lecture informative and usually entertaining. Paid WW lecturers are former fat people who have kept their weight off and gone through a training period. They know what they're talking about and are usually warm, enthusiastic, and, occasionally, dynamic. The class members have an opportunity to ask questions and share feelings, although not on the same level of confessionalism as Overeaters Anonymous. WW classes, the most accessible of The Big Four, are found in most towns and cities plus rural areas as well. Some places too small to boast their own movie theater have their own WW classes.

If you are interested in Weight Watchers, try several classes before you settle on one. The quality varies with the size of the class and the experience and personality of the lecturer. Do what's best for you.

Diet Workshop: This second largest of the franchise diet groups, with 63 area franchises and 1900 groups, may try harder than WW because it is number two. Diet Workshop group leaders are taught to take a personal interest in you when you come to a meeting. (You may be surprised by a telephone call, asking you to come back if you decide DW isn't for you.) The DW program is probably the most well-rounded of them all and includes a well-balanced diet (for men, women and teens), behavior modification, nutrition education and exercise. Complete menus and recipes round out the material offered newcomers.

"It's In to Be Thin," the DW motto, is certainly much on display in their group meetings. The bubbly, thin group leader gives a fount of information, a new diet recipe every week and encouragement for every member. Newcomers are offered a Four-Point Lifetime Weight Control booklet, called in computer-type parlance, Phase I. This booklet becomes your bible until you reach your weight goal, when you are given (you guessed it) the Phase II booklet to help you maintain your weight.

At each meeting, members are privately weighed and given an opportunity to share their problems and experiences. After your first meeting you'll receive an intensive briefing on the entire program so that you will have a goal and a means to reach it right from the start.

Like Weight Watchers, the Diet Workshop is a minimal expense for overweights, certainly less than many contract salons and probably much less than you spend on unneeded food per week.

146

There is a no-nonsense, modern (without being too sophisticated), comprehensive feeling about the DW approach. Group size is limited so that you can get the individual attention and recognition that most people (not just overweights) want. A Diet Workshop meeting is definitely one you should try before finding a diet group home.

Other Diet Groups of Note

Overeaters Victorious: The fast-growing fundamental religious movement has its own diet group in the form of Overeaters Victorious, not connected in any way with Overeaters Anonymous. Founded in late 1977 by Neva Coyle, a young Minnesota housewife, OV sells correspondence courses with lessons and teaching cassettes which may be ordered from the central office for less than $40. Thirty-two chapters were formed during OV's first year, all of them following a philosophy based on ancient Christian doctrine which states that answers to all problems can be found in the Bible.

Founder Coyle says she had done everything she could think of to lose weight, even submitting to an intestinal by-pass operation. Still 54 pounds overweight, she found a fat church friend and they decided to meet twice a week to help each other search the Bible for God's answer to overweight. "We prayed for each other," she says, "and searched scriptures for ways to stop eating. We couldn't find many references to overeating. What we *did* find were many scripture messages that promised victory."

The doctrine is simple, says Neva Coyle: "God is calling every overweight to be a responsible, controlled person and He holds us accountable for what we do with our bodies."

It's up to you. If Overeaters Victorious philosophy fits into your lifestyle, you may want to find out more about their plan by writing their address listed at the end of this chapter.

The Schick Program: Many Schick alcoholic and smokers' treatment centers, with their unique combination of aversion therapy and relaxation techniques, are also taking on weight-loss clients. Overweights are gradually induced to stop overeating, particularly on sweets, by being forced to watch themselves stuff in front of wall-to-wall mirrors while the odor of dead fish is piped into the room. Later, clients learn relaxation methods (by this time they need them) in order to help remove temptations.

My own opinion is that overweights suffer enough without deliberately exposing themselves to additional unpleasantness, but I have talked with overweights who swear by their Schick experience. Again, there are so many options open to you in diet groups, both self help and paid help (as Schick is), that you can find a perfect match for your needs. Costs can run to more than $250 on the Schick regimen.

Diet Consultants: This small, but growing, group (again in Minnesota), epitomizes the new wave in diet groups. They bring it all together in a total program for overweights which includes individualized attention and an all-important follow-up plan for maintainers. I'm impressed that this group with its holistic mind-body-emotions approach is the very best kind of group for overweights.

Psychological Group Therapy for Weight Loss

In almost every hamlet and burg there are therapy groups which help the overweight become more aware of the hefty habits that they must halt before they can keep weight off permanently. It's true that some people recognize these changes for themselves or in non-profit diet groups, but others need to go farther. *There is no stigma attached to getting psychological help for your overeating problem.* You're not "nuts." On the contrary, you're smart.

How can you find therapy groups for the overweight? Try asking your doctor, or if that's too embarrassing (doesn't he know you're fat?) call your county medical society and ask for a referral to a group specializing in your problem. Call the local YWCA or contact the hospital in your area that has a psychiatric out-patient clinic. Chances are you will find several choices in behavior therapy groups which will help you halt destructive eating habits.

The Un-diet Group

In the battle between the forces of largeness and the forces of smallness, NAAFA (National Association to Aid Fat Americans) has given as good as it's got, getting in quite a few strikes for the fat underdog. Not anti-diet, but not pro-diet either, NAAFA comes out roundly for free choice. This may be very hard for the thin-oriented overweight in the United States to understand, but there are some fat people who *want to stay fat.* So why don't they, without forming an organization and making a fuss?

The NAAFA people are fighters, that's why. They're the libbers of downtrodden overweights everywhere. Their purpose is to promote tolerance in society towards overweight human beings; and, bless them, they even believe that fat *can* be beautiful. They fight

148

against job discrimination, limited fashionable clothing in large sizes, low self-esteem and social stigma wherever they find it. They have chastized movie stars, admirals, millionaires, hotel chains and newspapers. In short, they are about the most assertive, self-respectful group for overweights around. They provide a dating service for their members which lists ideal weights to over 400 pounds, and they have women and men asking for this weight in a date. Their influence worldwide has caused similar groups to be founded in England and Japan.

Not many overweights in today's western culture can agree that fat is beautiful, but we all *must* agree that it is not ugly. It is a problem of body, mind and spirit, not of good or bad.

If you have lost and regained your weight many times, perhaps, as NAAFA and some health experts say, it is better to stabilize at a high weight than to continue on the fat-thin roller coaster, building up fat deposits in your arteries. If that's where you are, why not consider NAAFA for the support you'll need to live with your decision in a thin chauvinistic world? As for the rest of us, who long for a thinner, healthier lifestyle, the least we can do is support the NAAFA people with three cheers for luck.

Diet Groups and Your Holistic Plan

If holism has two absolutes, they are these: you have a right to all the help you need, but ultimately, getting thin and staying thin is your responsibility.

Diet groups can give acceptance and dignity to lives that have little of either. Many have been helped with one of the most curious and baffling problems of our modern age. But remember, while many are helped, some are hurt. Don't allow the fear of dropout guilt to hamper your recovery from the quicksand of overeating.

Each of us has an innate drive toward health. It is rooted in the center of our being and often can be unlocked by identification with a group of others like us. It is a strange phenomenon of this problem of ours that we can be helped by another fat man or woman when we may not be helped by experts in the field. It is for you to discover if diet self-help groups or group therapy are the key to your own life.

I have seen group action work miracles by releasing dormant energies and allowing a person literally to explode into activity. I have seen overweights find a home in their group to an almost mystical extent. At last, they think, we are accepted as we are. The group provides more than acceptance; it also makes it possible to acquire more discipline through the strength of many.

With this strength, added to your own inner but underdeveloped strength, you *can* acquire self-mastery and freedom from the dominance of the eons-old instinct to overeat. You *can* take control of your body, mind and spirit, building a solid highroad to well-being.

For so long, we overweights have shied away from the concept of self-control, thinking that the mere admission of the thought would cause guilt. After all, we ask ourselves, if we have it, why don't we use it? That is a negative viewpoint. First, we must learn that our natural ability to control ourselves is the absolute essence of freedom. Then, we will *want* to use it.

Group help may or may not be a component of your lifestyle assault on overweight. That is for you to decide, since all the power of decision rests in your hands. But decide you must, one way or the other, because, today, you are getting on with the business of living. As you read these lines, your body is sending you a message, a message that says it is sick and tired of feeling sick and tired. LISTEN. Then, read the next chapter. Don't be put off by the "dirty" word exercise. You will discover that there may be more in it for you than you ever realized.

Diet Group Registry

Diet Consultants, Suite 300, 12450 Wayzata Boulevard, Minnetonka, Minnesota 55343   Telephone (612) 546-8323

Diet Control Center, Inc., 1021 Stuyvesant Avenue, Union, New Jersey 07083   Telephone (201) 687-0007

Diet Workshop, Inc., 3375 Park Avenue, Wantagh, New York 11793   Telephone (516) 781-6207

National Association to Aid Fat Americans, (NAAFA), P.O. Box 43, Bellerose, New York 11426   Telephone (212) 776-8120

Overeaters Anonymous, World Service Office, 2190-190th Street, Torrance, California 90504   Telephone (213) 320-7941

Schick Centers, 1901 Avenue of the Stars, Suite 1530, Los Angeles, California 90067   Telephone (212) 553-9771

Take Off Pounds Sensibly, (TOPS), 4575 South 5th Street, P.O. Box 4489, Milwaukee, Wisconsin 53207

Weight Losers International, 5500 West Capitol Drive, Milwaukee, Wisconsin 53216   Telephone (414) 444-9100

Weight Watchers International, Inc., 800 Community Drive, Manhasset, New York 11030   Telephone (516) 627-9200

HOLISTIC LIFESTYLE CHANGE 10

I believe in giving myself every possible opportunity to win at the "weighting" game by:

1. Keeping an open mind about diet self-help groups.

2. Making an effort to match my personality to the right group.

3. Not feeling guilty if I want to leave a group for whatever reason.

4. Seeking psychological group therapy if other diet groups don't work for me, or if I prefer therapy in the first place.

5. Remembering that, while groups are important to my achieving an overall lifestyle change, the responsibility for thinness ultimately rests in the center of my being.

ARE YOU A COMPULSIVE OVEREATER?

		Yes	No
1.	Do you eat when you're not hungry?	☐	☐
2.	Do you go on eating binges for no apparent reason?	☐	☐
3.	Do you have feelings of guilt and remorse after overeating?	☐	☐
4.	Do you give too much time and thought to food?	☐	☐
5.	Do you look forward with pleasure and anticipation to the moments when you can eat alone?	☐	☐
6.	Do you plan these secret binges ahead of time?	☐	☐
7.	Do you eat sensibly before others and make up for it alone?	☐	☐
8.	Is your weight affecting the way you live your life?	☐	☐
9.	Have you tried to diet for a week (or longer), only to fall short of your goal?	☐	☐
10.	Do you resent the advice of others who tell you to "use a little will power" to stop overeating?	☐	☐
11.	Despite evidence to the contrary, have you continued to assert that you can diet "on your own" whenever you wish?	☐	☐
12.	Do you crave to eat at a definite time, day or night, other than meal time?	☐	☐
13.	Do you eat to escape from worries or trouble?	☐	☐

14. Has your physician ever treated you for overweight? ☐ ☐
15. Does your food obsession make you or others unhappy? ☐ ☐

How did you score? If you answered yes to three or more of these questions it is probable that you have a compulsive eating problem or are well on the way to having one.

DIET GROUP PERSONALITY CHECKLIST

Circle One

Yes No 1. I prefer the friendship of self-help group members to the distance of a psychologist or the anxiety of therapy group confrontation.

Yes No 2. I have feelings of isolation and alienation from my family and friends because of my weight problem.

Yes No 3. I feel I need more help than one person (husband/wife/friend) can give me.

Yes No 4. I am peer oriented. I like to get together with others who are like me.

Yes No 5. I feel better when I know others are concerned and are not "looking down on me."

Yes No 6. I am a confessional person. I like to talk with others in a frank way about my problems.

Yes No 7. I am not a confessional person. In a group, I can protect my anonymity if that is my wish.

Yes No 8. I am attracted to ideologies (Christianity, Republicanism, Behavior Modification).

Yes No 9. I always do better when I have competition.

Yes No 10. I feel good when someone else tells me that what I'm doing is right.

Yes No 11. I am a woman. (80% of diet group members are female.)

Yes No 12. I am a boy or girl between 13 and 18. (Peers are most important at this age.)

Yes No 13. I am more enthusiastic in a group than I am alone.

Yes No 14. I believe I can get more help from a person who has been fat than a person who has always been thin.

SCORING: If you answered seven or more questions with Yes, you might feel quite comfortable in a diet group of your choice.

Chapter Eleven

Exercise: the Ultimate Test of Self

Every morning, a woman I know very well pumps five miles on an Exercycle. At noon, she takes another two-mile bicycle ride around the neighborhood, following up in the late afternoon with a 50-lap performance in her pool. As often as not, she walks the dog (and her husband) after dinner. What kind of exercise nut is she? No exercise nut at all, but a formerly fat woman keeping herself in aggressively good health. As you may have guessed, the woman is me, but I don't find all that exercise exhausting. On the contrary, I find that I can do everything with more efficiency and verve when I get my body out from behind this typewriter and *move it*. It may sound trite, but a flexible body makes life better all around.

If you were a fat child, as I was, you probably hated exercise in school. Remember? The other kids never wanted you on their teams, and the teacher usually forced one side or the other to take you on. (To this day, I have an unrequited desire to teeter-totter because no one was heavy enough to be my partner on the playground see-saw!) In high school, most of us became physical education drop-outs, finally refusing to have anything more to do with the negative, embarrassing world of exercise. Temporarily defeated by demands on our bodies which we hadn't the self-esteem to fulfill, we fell back, some of us for decades, into a state of inanimate blobbery.

A male friend of mine who was a fat youngster recounts an all too familiar story from the man's viewpoint. "When it came to team sports, I was always unanimously chosen scorekeeper," he recalls, sarcastically. "But for me, gym classes were the worst. I was just unable to run as fast or do as many push-ups as the other fellows, and the punishment for that was to run extra laps and do push-ups after school. The whole thing was so punitive that for years after, I tried to stay as far away from all exercise as I could." This, from a well-built man who placed number one in an all-city tennis tournament for over thirty-fives.

If you had negative exercise-play experiences in childhood, your story is fairly typical of young overweights. But even if you didn't gain extra weight until you were an adult, physical exercise isn't all that attractive. "The truth is," says Richard Ecker, M.D. who specializes in exercise programs for the obese, "that exercise is physically harder for a fat person than a thin person." There! The doctor has confirmed your worst suspicions. It looks as if any form of physical exertion is just what you suspected — a particularly sadistic form of self-torture. Yes, you may think that, may truly believe that, but as you read on in this chapter you are going to discover the world of exercise *can* be a friendly place for overweights if you know what it's all about.

Making exercise a part of your lifestyle has nothing to do with feeling good or looking good — although they're two of the results. All the experts who try to motivate you by telling you these things are making a futile appeal. Truly, most fat men and women don't think they deserve to feel or look good.

What is the motivation *you* will need to get going on an exercise program and stick to it? Simply this: you will exercise to test your self-respect, to add to your own stature as a person, to give yourself more value in the scheme of your life. *Exercise is one big way you can prove yourself to yourself.*

No, I'm not going to lie to you. Your muscles will ache, your feet will be sore and you will feel tired — at first. And that's just the point where you always stopped your exercise program in the past, long before you got to the good part. This time you won't quit, because exercise will become a part of your respect for yourself.

Sure, it's going to take several days before you feel a lift in spirit, several weeks before you see a noticeable body change and maybe longer before you actually begin to improve your health. So don't expect your personal exercise effort to be the "Mt. Everest" of exercise programs. You are going to be reshaping and fine-tuning your body and it is going to take time, energy and commitment. What's the difference between this time and all the other times you thought you would like to get into shape? This time you have the self-esteem to work for your body. *This time you can take it.*

But it won't just be an exercise in moral and physical fortitude. Your efforts will have rewards, if you give yourself a healing chance. I won't promise you the body of an Adonis or the figure of Marilyn Monroe, but I will promise you one thing: you will be able to say to yourself, "I am playing the game to win." And incidentally, you are going to start feeling and looking great.

Holistically speaking, there is no question that body healing through exercise is an equal partner with emotional and spiritual healing. Health exists only so long as these three elements function well in harmony with each other. Disease occurs when one of these elements ceases to function.

What Is the Role of Exercise in Your Life?

I'm not going to try to scare you "for your own good" by telling you horror stories about sedentary lifestyles. Everybody today knows that people who don't get sufficient exercise are more prone to heart disease and a host of other problems. But let me tell you some of the benefits I and others have experienced, and then you make up your own mind based on your growing self-esteem.

1. Because I've developed a more efficient cardiovascular system, I have not only reduced the chance of heart disease, but I'm able to climb stairs, walk fast and carry things, all without huffing and puffing.

2. I lowered my blood pressure from 160/95 to 125/80, a near classic reading.

3. I discovered that I can control body fat better with exercise plus diet than with just diet alone. By exercising (moving continuously) for one-half hour every day, you will discover that you can be 26 pounds lighter after one year, all without changing your food intake. So you don't have an extra half-hour a day. Neither do I. I do other things while pedaling my Exercycle, like watching the morning news.

4. Doctors tell me I've slowed the aging process and have the internal organs of a woman ten years my junior.

5. I feel less stress and tension and, therefore, I don't want to overeat as often.

6. I have a day-to-day feeling of well-being, both physical and psychological. I have a sense of body-pride because I know I can stretch my muscles and *win*.

Grandpa Didn't Have to Jog

Don't you wish you lived a hundred years ago? There was no question of jogging or other artificial exercises to keep healthy. Almost everybody did hard, physical work. My farmer grandfather thought nothing of cutting a walking staff and tramping five miles over the hill to his apple orchard whenever he needed to inspect it. By the time he'd breakfasted at 7:30 each morning he had already exercised every muscle in his body for three hours.

But gradually modern machines and urban living made muscles less important and supplemental exercise more important. And as the majority of the western world's population became fatter and fatter, exercise became vital to health.

Wait a minute. You know that, don't you? Doesn't it follow that we overweights, as intelligent people, would begin to exercise as soon as we discovered our need. No, it doesn't follow. Why? Because as Dr. Ecker said, exercise is harder for us. On top of that, we have all those bad memories of gym class and we think that exercising isn't any fun. Damn it! Isn't life supposed to be fun, we ask?

We're in our now familiar Catch-22 situation again. We need to exercise because our lifestyle has had most of the natural exercise programmed out of it. On the other hand, we have been psychologically conditioned to blobbery and to believing that "if it's good for us, it ought to be instant, easy and fun."

Our world is geared to providing instant everything. If a television series doesn't make us laugh right now, it disappears. All new products are sold with the word EASY prominent in their advertising. New medical discoveries are touted as miracles. Our culture has taught us all, fat and thin alike, to expect instant, easy, fun miracles.

When it comes to exercise, this prevailing attitude doesn't hurt thin people nearly as much as it hurts us. Remember, exercise isn't as hard for them to accomplish. But it is for us, and too many of us have given up in the past when the going got tough. After all, we tell ourselves, if exercise isn't easy and fast, then it must not be good for us. BOSH! When I used such specious reasoning, my old grandfather used to say, "I'd like to buy you for how much you're worth, and sell you for how much you think you're worth." He gave me another grandfatherly moral: "Anything worth having, is worth working for." If your own elders gave you such advice, as they surely must have, don't shrug it off just yet. My hard-exercising, sinewy-muscled grandfather lived to be eighty-nine and never carried an extra pound of fat. He would never in the world understand how his granddaughter became imprisoned in a fat cell.

Exercise must be part of your lifestyle assault on obesity. If you think not, you are kidding yourself. Turn around and think about it again. Maybe exercise is more important to your successfully winning through to a thinner life than you imagined. Why don't you read on and see?

Exercise and the Obesity Connection

It's almost too much to believe, but some research has shown that obese people don't eat as much as thin people. The interesting thing is that thin people are *much* more active. Dr. Jean Mayer, the famed nutritionist, observed as long ago as 1955 that fat children in the same game with thin children managed to play with very little movement.

An old Chinese proverb states: Never do anything standing that you can do sitting, or anything sitting that you can do lying down. Most overweights have taken this proverb as their personal motto. Unfortunately such a slogan will lead not only to an unhealthy body but also to terminal boredom. Inactivity is the martyrdom of the physical body.

One of the great myths of exercise which we overweights cling to is that it makes us hungrier. Wrong again. Physical activity is an essential element in appetite control. When you do not exercise, your appetite doesn't function accurately. It can tell you to eat more calories than you have expended.

There is no greater proof that inactivity is at the root of obesity than in cattle raising. What do farmers do when they want to fatten cattle? They restrict the animal's activity by confining them in small areas, *where they can get no exercise.*

If you wanted to deliberately fatten yourself, the best prescription would be to confine yourself to as little exercise as possible with as much food as you could eat. If you want to un-fatten yourself, you would do the opposite. Obviously!

When you decide that your top priority is your whole body's health, when you really want to test yourself and come up a winner, when you really want to look and feel terrific, consistent exercise is one very important aspect you should consider incorporating into your lifestyle. It won't be easy, but it may not be as impossibly hard as you think. You may even find, as many have, more purpose for your existence when you have the full use of your own body.

You Don't Know It, but You're Already Exercising

One of the hardest things about exercise is getting enough motivation to start. What if, without knowing it, you had already started an exercise program? If you were already exercising, it stands to reason that you wouldn't have to begin, you would only need to extend and improve what you had already started. Take a good look at the chart on pages 172 and 173 labeled *Hidden Exercises*. Add your score and see how well you are doing without even knowing it.

Of course, you probably don't do, as I don't, many of these exercise activities for an hour or more a day, but by prorating the time I do spend, I discovered that I exercised away 365 calories a day. According to the experts, that means that if I ate only enough calories to maintain my weight, I would lose one pound every ten days *just in the course of my normal activities.* That's thirty-six pounds a year! Figure it out for yourself. Use 3,500 calories as the energy base for one pound and divide by the number of hidden exercise calories you expend every day. How long would it take for you to lose a pound? Ten pounds?

Movement Modification: Stretching Yourself a Little Bit

When I was a hundred pounds overweight, if someone had suggested I jog for exercise, I would have thought he or she was cruel, or stupid or funny, but not serious. What I *was* able to do was to stretch myself just a little, working those frozen joints and stiff muscles enough to get myself moving and limber again. From that moment, I stopped being a dead weight!

Stretch and Flex

1. **Arm Reach:** "Grab for the sky, podner," was good advice during an old western stage coach robbery and, today, for the general creakiness of unused upper limbs. Now, get up on your toes and stretch for the ceiling. Next stretch toward the walls. Finally, move your arms about in small circles, just a few times at first, then more later so you can exert a pull on flabby upper arms.

2. **Ball Game:** Keep a rubber ball by your telephone and while you're talking, clench it in your fist and relax, first one hand then the other.

3. **Head Roll:** Whenever you find yourself standing to do a job (and nobody's looking) roll your head around on your neck. It may snap, crackle and pop like a famous breakfast cereal. Don't worry. You won't hear a sound in a couple of days.

4. **Shoulder Shrug:** Roll your shoulders by rotating them in a shrug, one after the other.

5. **Telephone March:** While standing still or talking on the telephone, march to some imaginary music, lifting one leg as high as you can and then the other for some sneaky exercise and limbering movements.

6. **Foot Fun:** While sitting, take off your shoes and stockings, place your toes at the edge of your telephone book and grasp it then release. This helps to exercise your feet so they won't quit when you need them most.

7. **No-water Swimming:** Bend at the waist with feet wide apart and make swimming movements with both arms, swinging them in front of you and then behind as if you were doing the Australian crawl.

You'll want to give yourself a self-massage after you've exercised, even these little stretch and flex activities. Think of your body as your good friend. You are doing whatever you can to relax the bodily tension and tiredness that often builds up during a hectic day.

Tell yourself after every exercise session that you love yourself. Wrap your arms around your body and sway back and forth in an easy rhythm — just you and your body. Breathe in and breathe out, deeply and slowly. If you make any exercise, no matter how minor, a quiet, joyful time (no sweating or groaning just yet, please), you will be more apt to approach the next step with some eagerness, a sense of potential pleasure and that all-important sense of winning accomplishment.

Inner Exercises

Before you can make the big switch from placidity to strength you need to accomplish two things:

1. Check with your doctor to see that you are physically capable of exercising. It's the truly rare overweight who can't expend some energy.

2. Get yourself into the proper mental mood.

Research at the University of California discovered that many obese people in their exercise programs had "depersonalized" their bodies. In other words, there were parts they didn't use, didn't even seem to want to "own." The result was that these parts were moved very little, even when the owners thought they were exercising. Sometimes fat people don't like to move, researchers say, because they think they might lose control of their bodies. They can be really afraid of fast movement for this reason. It would be wrong for that person literally to jump into a strenuous program of tennis. Instead, very gradual exercises of simple movements are prescribed which involve every part of the body. They begin on a chair, then move to the floor, using the wall for support, and finally graduate to real energy expenditure.

If you are feeling such body-distrust, you may need to go back over the body-awareness exercises in Chapter Five before you can come again to physical exercise. One of the reasons, I believe, why so many overweights are exercise drop-outs is that they have such a dislike (even distaste) for their bodies that they simply don't want to work with them in any way. "It appears," says psychologist Michael Murphy, "that the body is not so much the end of (exercise) as the beginning."

Your body is your centering point, your place to start from. If you have a feeling of love and regard for your body it will be a sturdy base for reaching *beyond* everything of which you think you are now capable. Exercise, for you, will not be an end in itself, but the beginning of an unfolding of your human potential that will eventually extend the boundaries of your lifestyle.

Remember the last time you went for a picnic with your family or friends? When the others wanted to explore, you stayed behind with the picnic basket, saying, "You go ahead and I'll be here when you get back." From today, you will begin to change the way you use your body. You will play the game to win. You will begin to move. *You are on the move.*

Your Exercise Goals

When you start a diet, you have a weight goal. It is just as logical to have Fitness Objectives when you start to exercise. Ask yourself: What do I want to accomplish by exercising? Probably number one on your *want list* is the hope that exercise will help you lose weight, which it will surely do. Number two may be to increase your stamina and improve your general physical health. Number three will certainly have something to do with improving your self-esteem, with passing a test you set for youself, with deciding to do something and not finding your resolve wanting.

Write down your personal Fitness Objectives on a piece of paper and whenever you feel sore, tired or sorry for yourself during the first few days of your exercise program, take out this piece of paper and refer to it. It will remind you that you have a purpose.

The next question (now that you're ready to begin) is what kind of exercise should you choose?

1. Will this exercise keep you moving, working you 70 or 85 percent of your maximum heart rate? Figure your maximum heart rate at 220 minus your age.

2. Can you eventually do this exercise for from 15 to 60 minutes a day?

3. Will you be able to participate in this exercise three to five days a week?

4. Is this an exercise that you can readily understand?

There are four basic types of exercises from which you can choose:

Isometrics: The object of isometric exercise is to promote muscular strength and bulk through contractions. This is accomplished by pushing or pulling against an immovable object, such as a door frame, or by pitting one group of muscles against another, which will give you the same effect.

Isotonics: These exercises are just a modern name for old fashioned toe touches, push-ups and sit-ups, which your high school gym teacher called calisthenics. They serve mainly to limber up or to condition the body. Weight lifting and not-too-active sports such as shuffle board and pitching horseshoes are isotonic exercises.

Anaerobics: A fifty-yard dash is a good example of this exercise, which is used to build endurance and stamina.

Aerobics: This physical activity increases heart and respiratory action for a sustained period of time, sending oxygen through the body and brain. Running, jumping rope, cycling, swimming and paddle ball all fall into this category of exercise.

Which of these exercise groups will prove most beneficial for you? Dr. Richard Ecker takes the guesswork out of your decision. "It's all right, of course, to participate in many kinds of exercise, but if you want to burn fat, you have to be aerobic." Why? Because aerobic exercise keeps you moving continuously and helps you produce your maximum ideal heart rate, for best cardiovascular and weight-losing results.

We won't go into the world of aerobic exercise in a scientific way here. Everything you want to know about aerobics can be answered by Dr. Kenneth Cooper in his runaway best seller books *Aerobics, New Aerobics* and *The Aerobics Way.* Read them. You will learn what physical activity can do to improve your body and your life.

Warm-up and Cool-out

No doubt, your fitness level is fairly low at this point, but even when it is very high don't forget that you must sandwich your exercise sessions with a warm-up and a cool-out.

Take at least five minutes before you begin sustained exercise to perform a series of stretches which will get your body prepared for what is to come. Likewise, after vigorous exercise you can feel light headed because blood is pooling in your legs. Again you need a three-to-five minute period of cooling-out with mild slowing-down exercises.

Don't Go at It Too Hard — Ever

Being a little on the compulsive side, we overweights usually start anything new at top speed. From now on, whenever you are exercising there is a rule of thumb for you to use so that you don't overdo. Ask yourself:

1. Am I pain-free?
2. Can I hold a conversation while exercising?

Unless you can answer both of these questions affirmatively, you are exercising too hard. LET UP.

Growing Strong

Here is a mini-encyclopedia of winning exercises you can choose. You may want to sample them smorgasbord-style until you discover one that really suits you. Look at the Calorie Equivalency Chart on page 173. You may want to concentrate on one now and move on to others later or you may want to simplify the entire process and choose the most popular exercise for overweights (with both experts and individuals) right from the start.

Walking

Did you guess that walking is probably the best all-around exercise for you? Isn't it amusing that for decades we have been told to get out and walk, but it may take scientific research to convince us?

Although there are dozens of studies, I'll mention only one here since they tend to duplicate results. The *American Journal of Clinical Nutrition* reported that one group of overweight women on a regimen of moderate diet and brisk walking for 17 weeks lost five percent of their body fat in that time. Moreover, their heart rate improved and their self-confidence zoomed along with an increased capacity for physical work. In other words, increased physical activity paradoxically created in them the ability to further increase physical activity.

Walking is especially good for women over 35 years old because they were of a generation conditioned to think exercise unladylike.

Women under 35 and men generally tend to accept other forms of exercise more readily.

Are you ready to begin walking? There's still one further hurdle to leap before you can really get into it. It is those saboteurs again, wanting to "help you." A friend of mine, who began a walking program in her neighborhood, finally had to get in her car and drive to a distant neighborhood for her daily walks. "My friends and neighbors had never seen me walking," she said, "and they all came out of their houses, thinking I needed a ride. I couldn't get any walking done."

When you begin to walk, place is important. Frankly, I got tired of walking the same blocks day after day, so I laid out several courses that took me thirty minutes to cover. One day I would walk through a nearby shopping center doing some window-shopping while I got my exercise; another day I'd walk in a park near my house, and another in the neighborhood school yard where I practiced my hopscotch whether anyone was looking or not.

You may want to follow Dr. Joyce Brothers' recommendation and walk with a purpose. If you can collect insects or plant specimens or are a bird watcher, walking can add to your collection and collection can add to your walking. I am an amateur landscaping buff so my walks provide me with ideas for new plant arrangements.

When you begin to walk, time is important. If you wait until you *find* time, you will never start. If you want time to do anything, you must *make* it. You should "make" at least thirty minutes a day, at least four times a week for a brisk walk. Although researchers say you can get benefits from walking (or indeed any exercise) as little as three times a week, significant weight loss usually occurs only at the four times or more a week level.

Walking one mile a day for one year can amount to a loss of over ten pounds a year. Dr. Barbara Edelstein, author of *The Woman Doctor's Diet for Women* goes further when she tells slow-losing older women who walk that they "can lose weight the way you did when you were thirty."

For many reasons, walking is the best exercise for the over-weight:

1. You can do it alone.
2. You can lose weight with or without a diet. (It just takes twice as long without a reduction in food intake.)

3. You can walk when you may not be able to jog or run.

4. You can do it anytime, anyplace. (It's hard to pack a bicycle for vacations or holidays.)

5. Unlike bicycling or swimming, when you walk you carry all your own weight. The more you weigh, the better walking is for you because you'll burn more calories than a thinner person.

6. It's inexpensive. You won't need any special equipment.

If you'd like to learn all there is to know about walking and then some, read Consumer Guide's *The Complete Book of Walking*, the book that turns ordinary walking into a sport.

Come on. Try walking. In this world where most of us dash around in cars all day, sitting above the earth, looking at it through plate glass windshields, we can sometimes lose touch with earthly reality. Walking brings you back to your personal connection with the planet, with its plant and animal life. You will find yourself seeing the smaller picture as you walk, bulbs pushing out of the ground, birds nesting, a moss-covered rock. It is uncommonly peaceful and more satisfying than a seven-course dinner.

"Above all, do not lose your desire to walk," wrote the troubled, crippled Danish philosopher Soren Kierkegaard. "Every day I walk myself into a state of well-being and walk away from every illness; I have walked myself into my best thoughts, and I know of no thought so burdensome that one cannot walk away from it."

Bicycling

Next on your list of great ways for overweights to exercise should be bicycling. It was the first exercise I tried once I got off my typewriter chair and made a commitment to exercise and self-worth.

My first bicycle was a third-hand, ill-painted set of wheels that rode like an overland truck. At first I envied those fancy ten-speeds, their fenders gleaming in the sun, but I soon came to realise that my sorry old one-speed was giving me the best workout I was likely to get on any bicycle. In two weeks, my legs were noticeably stronger and huffing and puffing a bad memory of the old days before exercise. I persuaded a friend to join me and our daily coffee klatch on wheels became one of the fun parts of my day. Best of all, I burned over 200 calories during my half-hour jaunt and gave myself a good aerobic workout.

You may prefer a stationary bike, either an Exercycle or a stand that lifts your rear wheel off the floor and turns a regular bicycle into an exercise machine. I have an Exercycle for inclement weather that I bought for $22 at a garage sale. (You can find much cast-off exercise equipment at garage or flea market sales.) Since Exercycling is a bit boring, I always try to use it while watching television or listening to a favorite record.

My ultimate Exercycle fantasy is to buy a Dynavit, a space-age exercise bicycle with a built-in computer that does about everything but figure your income tax. The Dynavit can be programmed with your weight and age, then gives you a continuous readout *(while you're cycling)* of ideal heart rate and how many calories you're expending. No guesswork here! (If you want to know more, contact Dynavit of America, 305 Era Drive, Northbrook, Illinois 60062.)

Jogging and Running

Jogging or running may not be the best exercise for you, if you are very much overweight. All that weight, and all that pounding — 800 footfalls a mile — may put too much stress and strain on your legs and feet. If you're not extremely overweight and your doctor okays a jog-run program, you may want to consider taping your ankles (ask a high school coach or nurse how to do this) and you might want to have a custom-made arch support for your special sport shoes.

Attention Women! Since jogging reduces fat deposits, you may not want to consider it if your breasts are too small to begin with. Breasts are made of fat and skin and some women joggers have complained of losing breast size when seriously jogging.

Jogging or running is usually an exercise to which you can graduate after losing some weight and increasing your aerobic fitness. It has many benefits, according to afficionados. You can rapidly reach high fitness levels and maintain them, lose weight and even reach a kind of psychological euphoria where solutions to life's problems come easier. Most joggers and runners surveyed take better care of their health than nonrunners, eat more natural foods, and smoke and drink less. They even report fewer illnesses which require going to bed.

It is a great sport-exercise, and about 15 percent of all people who exercise choose jogging or running or a combination of the two. Nevertheless, for overweights, it can be embarrassing until we firm up in other ways. As one woman said: "When I run, *everything* moves!"

Swimming

Water is the great equalizer. When you are swimming, you are not old or young, thin or fat: you are in *your* element. You may not jog, run, walk or bicycle as fast as others, but you can swim as well. Why? Because when you're submerged in water you lose 90 percent of your weight. That means if you weight 150 pounds on dry land, you're a svelte 15-pounder in the water.

It's a good thing to swim before a meal, not because you may get stomach cramps if you swim after, but because exercise before a meal releases a hormone into your blood stream which decreases your appetite. If you really go all out, as I do by swimming laps for calorie expenditure, you can burn up your next meal before you eat it.

Swimming uses every muscle in the body *while providing a natural support for your body weight.* If you have any problems with your knees, feet or back, swimming is a fine way of exercising and strengthening them without putting stress on them. It is a great psychological exercise, too, since submerging your body in water is probably the most relaxing thing you can do to it. You will literally wash away tension.

Aerobically, swimming makes your heart work, and work hard, in a continuous and controlled manner, depending on how fast you stroke.

I have a strong tendency to want to use a pool like a giant bath tub. I love to sit on the steps and splash water on my shoulders, float around looking at clouds, in other words, "bathe" more than swim. I have to force myself to swim laps every spring, starting at ten laps and working up to fifty laps which takes me approximately thirty minutes at a steady pace.

Now, a word about the one drawback to swimming — the anguish and humiliation we can feel at appearing at the water in a bathing suit. But be practical and take a good look around you when you feel this way. How many wonderful bodies do you see on anyone over the age of twenty? Not many. *Your body* has as much right to exercise as any other body. You are a beautiful human being moving toward an integrated life. Don't drag yourself around the pool or beach as if you had something to be ashamed of. You have every reason to be proud of yourself.

The U.S. Government Printing Office puts out a marvelous booklet on physical conditioning through water exercise called *Aqua*

Dynamics. You can get a copy for yourself by writing The President's Council On Physical Fitness and Sports, Washington, D.C., 20201.

Dancercize

"Can you believe it? She's so light on her feet." I used to hear them whisper in amazement as I danced by and, indeed, I believe there are truly many fat people who move with great ease, play games like basketball, tennis or dance like a ballroom whiz. If you're one of these, you may want to take advantage of a new craze called dancercize, which is really exercise with some pizzazz in it. Classes in dance studios and in adult education programs are popping up everywhere, and you can even do it, as they say, in the privacy of your own home.

Dancercize (or if you prefer Exerdance) is very aerobic because it keeps you moving in time to the music. It's best to play the music loud, says Bonnie Prudden, famed exercise expert. "Music takes away a person's inhibitions," she explains. "When it's loud, the exerciser isn't thinking about how she looks. The music takes over and blocks out all those self-conscious feelings." You can work up a good "high" in dancing because you tend to exert more with less conscious effort.

Did you enjoy the body awareness exercise "Dance With Your Body" in Chapter Five? If you did, you'd probably like dancing as exercise. Again, it takes very little equipment, just you and a radio or phonograph.

Of all the exercises in this chapter, dancing is probably the one that answers the most basic human need for physical expression. (It's mentally healthy, too.) Think about it. There is something wild, even primitive, about dancing that's tied into the human experience. It frees your emotions, especially when you can accompany yourself with hand clapping, foot stomping and even shouting. It is truly body, mind, spirit holistic exercise.

If you want to know more about dance exercise, get the paperback book *Jazzercise* by Judy Sheppard Missett and Donna Meilach.

Jump-for-Fitness

An interesting alternative (or addition) to all the exercises mentioned above is jumping rope. It's not just a kid's game anymore. It requires a little space, a short piece of rope and a soft jumping surface. (Don't make the mistake of jumping on concrete, as I did, or you'll get absolutely hellish shin-splints.)

Rope jumping does your cardiovascular system as much good as jogging and gives you fast results you can see and feel within two weeks. Jumping 15 minutes a day is equivalent to three sets of tennis, 27 holes of golf or 20 minutes of swimming. According to one diet doctor, *two minutes a day* is the same as walking a mile.

Why aren't more people doing it? It is a hard exercise for overweights, but if you can work up to it with other conditioning exercises, it is the best get-it-over-with-quick way to fitness you will ever find.

Go easy on this one, but try it. You may be surprised at what you can do.

A Word of Caution About Exercise Salons

"If you're size 16 today, you can be size 10 by Christmas!"

"Hurry! Half-price special. Bring a friend. Two join for the price of one!"

"Lose 20 pounds or more in just 10 days on our special machines!"

When you make an exercise decision to exchange your tired body for a new lease on living, you may be attracted to such "exclamation point advertising" as the above. The physical fitness industry is an exploding business these days, taking advantage of our raised national weight and physical fitness consciousness. Don't get me wrong. On the whole, health spas, gyms and salons are legitimate business enterprises, and will help you exercise if you need someone to help you or are fascinated by the array of chrome machines offered in most health palaces. There is absolutely nothing wrong with joining a salon, if you want to spend the money and know what you're getting into.

1. Before you sign on for any health or weight-loss program at a salon, discuss your plans with your doctor and show him a copy of the diet and exercise regimen the salon offers.

2. Go to the salon and inspect the premises during their busiest times (mornings and after work) so you can see if they have enough equipment to accommodate all the people they have under contract.

3. Don't sign a contract during the inspection visit, no matter how much you are pressured to do so. Take a good look at the personnel, too. Are they extremely young and inexperienced? I could

be accused of being anti-youth, but I resent being advised on diet and exercise by a very young woman who knows little about either and calls me "honey" in a patronizing way.

4. Is the equipment active or passive? In other words, do you have to work it or does it work you? Most of the experts agree that passive vibrating rollers, belts and tables are pleasant but ineffective.

5. Try to talk to other salon members about their experiences.

6. Avoid lifetime membership contracts unless you have a track record of devotion to physical fitness. Some salons try to sell you such contracts, knowing that you will probably drop out. If possible, buy the shortest and cheapest membership you can until you decide if this is truly the way you want to handle your exercise program.

7. Don't allow yourself to be pressured by embarrassment. One disillusioned spa patron told me her free figure analysis turned out to be embarrassing exercises in front of a full-length mirror with others looking on. "I would have signed *anything*," she said, "just to get out of there."

You can't be too cautious. Contracts are binding legal agreements. If you drop out and refuse to pay, you can be sued. Newspapers reported that Jack LaLanne spas sued more than 650 clients in New York City alone during a recent year. Not only would a lawsuit wreck your mood and your credit record but probably your exercise program as well.

Visit several health and weight-reduction salons. If you like a no-nonsense physical fitness approach, the too-social salon might not be right for you. If you want something more folksy, there are many spas where you'd feel right at home. Match the salon to your own personality.

There are super-spas which are havens for the shape-up vacation crowd. You can get six hours of exercise, luxurious massages, secret spice wraps, whirlpool and steam baths plus miniscule meals for as little as $100 or as much as $1000 a day. If you ever suddenly come into an inheritance from old Uncle Harry, you may want to try exercising beautiful-people style. See page 171 for a list of fabulous exercise spas.

Exercise and Your Holistic Lifestyle

The holistic healer developing in you looks at your whole body and tries to see what can be found to improve it. This healer at your center wants to communicate with you about your body, wants to send you body signals which you will need to be able to monitor.

Without exercise you may have a poor work attitude, much strain and tension, a lack of joint flexibility and chronic fatigue. All of these signals are being sent to you over and over and will continue to be sent until you assume responsibility (not guilt) for your body's fitness. Believe that exercise is your partner in holistic harmony, that it will help reduce the tension that accompanies the negative emotional condition of overweight. Believe that it will relax you more than nibbling will.

Exercise will help you in two rather paradoxical ways: it will focus your tremendous, bursting energy to live and it will provide you with a core of inner calm, the kind that enables great athletes to go beyond their own purely physical resources. The heightened consciousness you will experience as you get your body moving is important in developing a winning spirit. Oh sure, you are going to feel good and look better but, although it's hard for you to believe at this point, even more important to you will be the knowledge that exercise will validate your sense of your own worth. You will have tested yourself and won. The heaviest burden for us overweights is not the extra pounds no matter how many of them there are; the heaviest burden is the horrible thought that we have no value. By accepting the responsibility to exercise our bodies, we prove to ourselves beyond a doubt that we can walk tall. We can take it. We overweights can excel. We prove we can care about our bodies and listen carefully to our inner healer.

You may not be able to get into shape overnight. Fitness success, after all, isn't a flashy burst of activity. Success in anything, as the philosopher says, consists of a series of little daily victories. Here's to you and your victory-a-day exercise program.

If you are overweight, you have a 40 percent chance of having an overweight child. If your mate is also overweight the odds double to 80 percent. There is a special guilt an overweight parent feels when she or he sees a beloved child suffering the same discrimination they themselves once experienced. But your hands aren't tied. There are ways you can help your youngster and yourself, too. You will find this help in the next chapter.

■┼┼┼┼┼■────────0

Super Exercise Vacation and Diet Spas

East

Renaissance Revitalization Center, P.O. Box N4854, Cable Beach, Nassau, Bahamas   Telephone (809) 327-8441

Spa Fontainbleau, 4441 Collins Avenue, Miami, Florida 33140   Telephone toll free (800) 327-8360

Greenbrier, White Sulphur Springs, West Virginia 24986   Telephone toll free (800) 624-6070

Harbor Island Spa, 7900 Harbor Island, Miami Beach, Florida 33141   Telephone toll free (800) 327-7510

Institute for Physical Fitness, Prospect Toll Road, Stockbridge, Massachusetts 01262   Telephone (413) 298-3066

Hippocrates Health Institute, 25 Exeter Street, Boston, Massachusetts 02116   Telephone (617) 267-9525

West

Maine Chance, 5830 East Jean Avenue, Phoenix, Arizona 85018   Telephone (602) 947-6365

The Golden Door, Box 1567, Escondido, California 92025   Telephone (714) 438-9111

Rancho La Puerta, Tecate, California 92080   Telephone (714) 478-5400

171

HOLISTIC LIFESTYLE CHANGE 11

I will make copies of the following chart and complete them for each week until I no longer need them to exercise.

Self-rating Activity/Exercise Chart

Day	Hidden Exercises		Planned Exercises*	
	How long	Calories Used	How long	Calories Used
Monday				
Tuesday				
Wednesday				
Thursday				
Friday				
Saturday				
Sunday				

*Circle Yes or No

Yes	No	I accomplished at least one planned exercise four times this week. (Hidden exercises don't count).
Yes	No	I exercised a full thirty minutes each day.**

**Use the first week to build to thirty minutes, starting at ten minutes per exercise period and building to thirty minutes.

Hidden Exercise Chart

Exercise	Calories Expended Per Hour
Walking slowly	115-200
Light housework	115-200
Light gardening	125-200
Sewing	130
Writing letters	110
Sitting	100
Standing	100
Dressing and undressing	30-40
Ironing	160
Dishwashing	160
Eating	100
Cooking	170
Playing Piano	150

Typing	130
Taking a bath	160
General office work	150
Singing	75
Brushing teeth or hair	100
Answering telephone	50
Reading	25
Watching television	25
Driving an automobile	120

MY DAILY SCORE

Exercise to Calorie Equivalancy Chart*

Exercise	Calories Used Per Hour
Walking slowly	200
Walking fast	350
Jogging	800
Swimming	750
Bicycling slow	210
Bicycling fast	450
Roller skating	350
Ping Pong	360
Tennis Singles	450
Tennis Doubles	350
Skiing	600
Running	900
Squash or Handball	550
Vigorous calisthenics	550
Bowling	260
Golf	250
Climbing	800

*Energy expenditure for 150-pound person. Add calories for heavier person, subtract for lighter person.

Chapter Twelve

Parenting Overweight Children

Fatty, fatty two-by-four,
Can't get through the kitchen door . . .

This cruel song echoes through thousands of school play-grounds. Each taunting refrain represents a lonely, emotionally-battered, fat child. That is sad enough, but quite often behind the fat child stands a grieving, guilt-ridden fat parent. "Talk about feeling guilty," exclaimed one mother, "it was more painful for me to see my daughter get fat than it was for me to be fat myself!" This anguished parent knew her child could be headed for a fat cell — a smaller one, true, but just as much a prison — unless this child was helped.

Obesity, now troubling the majority of adults, also affects more youngsters than ever before. A recent survey of Boston school children conducted by Harvard University's school of health turned up 20 percent as overfat — double the number reported twenty years earlier. How can parents keep their children from being mired in the quicksand of fat heredity? What, exactly, are parents to do?

First, don't feel guilty. Children gain weight for much of the same reasons that adults do — genetic, environmental, metabolic, psychological and, if female, because of sex. After taking reason-able precautions, such as serving nutritious food, creating a happy home atmosphere, accepting the child regardless of size and set-ting the best self-respectful example you can (all of which we'll get into in more depth later in this chapter), blaming yourself for your child's fat is like blaming yourself for giving him or her blue eyes. On the contrary, because you the parent are overweight, you can give your child special understanding no thin parent can give.

Second, make sure your child is really overweight, and that his or her "fat" is not just the result of your anxious imagination. If you have any doubts, use the skinfold or pinch test. The test works like this: Place the child's arm, hands down, in a relaxed position. Gently pinch up a fold a skin and fat tissue midpoint between shoulder and elbow on the backside of the arm without picking up the muscle. If the skinfold is over an inch thick, the child is over-weight.

In most cases the pinch test is unnecessary. Most of us know that our children are overweight when they are. How could this have happened to them? To us?

Why Children Gain Too Much Weight in Today's World

It is likely that adolescent outpatient clinics see more children with acne than any other problem. Isn't that right? No. This com-mon childhood complaint isn't number one, according to a national survey of adolescent medicine published in the *Delaware Medical Journal.* You guessed it. The primary, class A, numero uno prob-lem with teens is obesity.

Fortunately, if your child is obese the chance of its being caused by some physical illness is only one percent, but since even this small percentage represents thousands of children, you should be aware of the various possibilities.

Endocrine problems for your child need to be ruled out by a pediatrician, especially if the child is short for his or her age. Dr. C.B. Kim reported in the *Journal of the Indiana State Medical Association* that obesity in the short child is most likely to be related to endocrine balance.

A peculiar fat distribution, accompanied by bone retardation, skin and hair abnormalities can point to other physical problems named after their various discoverers such as Prader-Willi syn-drome, Froehlich syndrome, Laurence-Moon-Biedl syndrome and Pickwickian syndrome. These can be identified with laboratory testing. Dr. Kim confirms, however, that the overwhelming major-ity of obesity in children is due to overeating.

A very real problem for obese children that parents can active-ly combat is SUGAR. Mothers, especially fat mothers, have been the butt of criticism for years because we have been known to slip our kids a cookie. But that doesn't make mothers the all-time worst Cookie Monster. It is time to look at an even bigger culprit than mom. TELEVISION.

During one (interminable) four hour Saturday morning, I watched children's television and counted a total of 32 out of 59 commercials touting junk food. There were ads for cookies, candy bars, fast-food chains, altogether enough carbohydrates to supply the minimum daily requirement for the United States Army. Any child (or adult, for that matter) who watches this sugar assault week after week risks "diabetes of the eyes" as well as a galloping case of obesity.

Since the mid-1970's, complaints from chidren's groups have lowered the level of violence on some television programming aimed at youngsters, but little has been done about the *other* harmful message aimed at our already too-fat kids — EAT! EAT! EAT! (The Earth Mother deserves an Emmy for effective children's junk food programming.)

Is television food advertising more harmful for overweight youngsters than for slim ones? Yes, say researchers at the University of California at Davis. They showed some sugar snack slides to both groups, then asked the subjects to rate the products. Overweight kids rated the food higher after having seen slides than did the average-weight children.

The gnawing problem of too much sugar in young diets has even raised controversy in the schools where nonnutritious lunches and snacks account for a huge consumption of sugar-laden foods. In Burlington, Wisconsin all vending machines were removed from junior and senior high schools. In West Virginia (my former home state, usually considered educationally backward), the department of education recently forbade the sale of candy, gum, flavored ice bars and soft drinks in public schools. But this is only a carrot thrown to the anti-junk food forces, since the sale of sugar-flavored foods in this country's schools amounts to a $407 million industry.

It's sad when overweight youngsters who want to make right choices have hot lunch options that range from starchy-sugary school lunches to starchy-sugary snack meals at nearby food machines — in fact, no option at all.

Parents who are soured on sugar *can* make the difference. In Bloomington, Indiana a mother of four, backed by the local dental society and the PTA, had school vending machines restocked with fruits, nuts, yogurt and fruit juices. Other PTA's are renting their own machines offering nutritional foods.

Combat in the sugar zone takes on even more significance when parents, teachers and medical researchers show that a junk food diet is hard on a child in an emotional way. They can become aggressive, antisocial and depressed. Psychiatrist Richard Mackarness confirms this: "A diet full of starches and refined sugars simply does not provide enough energy to satisfy a child's bodily needs. So he is always hungry — and this hunger manifests itself in feelings of restlessness, agitation and bad temper." *What an added burden to place on the sagging shoulders of already oppressed fat children!*

Overweight children experience all the psychological buffeting that adults feel. They have disturbed body images long before they become adolescents. At Purdue University fat little five-year-olds were asked to choose the nicest silhouette of three. They all picked the thinnest one. It's heartbreaking to think that even such little ones have begun the culturally induced process of self-rejection.

Despite evidence to the contrary, overweight parents sometimes have trouble accepting the fat of their own flesh and blood. All too often they hope (and pray) that the problem will just go away in time. "When she begins to look at the boys, the pounds will come rolling off," my own plump mother used to say defensively when friends or relatives commented. "He'll lose it when he starts playing football in high school," many dads say hopefully. The tragic truth is quite different from that painted in these hopeful scenarios. The fat adolescent girl is a social outcast; the fat teenage boy has long since lost the desire to exercise.

The same sabotaging ridicule you experience will be the lot of your overweight child, forcing him or her to withdraw into fantasy (and food) or become the jolly clown. "I had to be a clown," said one man of his obese boyhood. "I was too fat to run and too scared to fight." Recalls Kathy: "Every night I prayed to God I'd wake up thin."

Recognizing the Two Danger Areas

There are two periods in a child's life when fat cells form most readily — between birth and two years and again from about eight to sixteen years. These are two times in your child's life when you *must* give his or her weight the most attention because, as you know, fat cells once formed can be reduced in size but never eliminated altogether. If a child gains an appreciable amount of weight during these danger years, they can accumulate as many as *six times* their normal quota of fat cells. An ounce of prevention during these years is worth many pounds of cure later.

Happily, the earliest danger period can be almost completely controlled by watchful parents. Here's how:

1. Breast feed, if you can. There is some evidence (and it's growing) that bottle-fed babies tend to eat too much simply

because there is a natural tendency for parents to want the child to "drink the whole thing." In other words, the bottle itself acts as a portion control rather than the baby's real hunger.

2. As insurance against forming too many fat cells, don't push your pediatrician into early solid feeding. Some doctors even recommend waiting six months before beginning fruit and cereal as long as vitamin supplements are adequate.

3. When solid feeding begins, don't use the manufacturer's container as a portion control. Many children don't want the whole jar.

4. If, in spite of these precautions, your baby has too many chins, the doctor can put him or her on a diet. This is the only time when you will have full control of what goes into your baby's mouth.

The next danger age, from eight to sixteen, presents different, and more complex, problems for you and for your child. Since there are so many positive ways you can help adolescents, we take those up in some depth later in this chapter.

What you are doing is perhaps more important than even you realize. You are attempting to break a genetic chain which has forged this cycle of familial obesity. You are extending a genealogical health gift not just to your progeny but to theirs, and all the generations of your blood and name to follow.

Your Overweight Child and the Doctor

It is just as important for your overweight child to have a positive experience with a physician as it is for you to have one. All the rules from Chapter Eight apply to your child. Overweight, after infancy, becomes much more than diet, medication and exercise prescriptions. The child needs to have help in building self-confidence, realizing that he or she is a valuable person and capable of losing weight. A doctor who doesn't treat a youngster as a whole child worthy of respect can do more damage than good. Choose your child's medical helper as you would your own.

One of the top experts on childhood obesity is Platon J. Collipp, M.D., pediatrician-in-chief of New York's Nassau County Medical Center. This doctor sets a high standard for medical treatment of the overweight child against which you can measure your own child's care. These are some discoveries he's made in the course of his practice.

1. Does the child *want* help? Dr. Collipp asks this question first, since a resentful child is difficult to approach.

2. Does the parent want help for the child? If not, says the doctor, childhood obesity is almost impossible to treat.

3. Weekly visits are best.

4. Agree on a goal, at the outset. "Children have to know where they're going, how long it's going to take," says the doctor, "or somewhere along the way they turn around and start back."

5. A two pound a week weight loss is average for his patients.

6. Dr. Collipp asks one question of his young patients each week. "What have you eaten that was not on your diet?" The only acceptable answer, he says, is *nothing.* "I give no praise or smile for eating. I only ask, 'why did you eat it?' " Unfortunately, according to the doctor, most children say their parents gave them permission to cheat. This is not always the parents' fault, reassures Collipp, because youngsters, especially teenagers, often manipulate parents into answers they are unaware are wrong.

7. Children are weighed every week. They need to know what they're losing, just as you do, and they need their goal reinforced at this time. At these weigh-ins, the doctor frequently adjusts food type and quantity to further personalize the child's diet.

8. Children can have snacks on diets. If a child is accustomed to snacks after school and in the evening, parents are advised to have snacks ready. Dr. Collipp even advises parents to let children know what snacks will be available upon their return from school. In this way the child can *plan* for them, without fantasizing inappropriate snacks. Acceptable snacking foods are low-calorie sodas, bouillon, fruit, low-calorie gelatin and salad vegetables.

9. Group therapy is good for most children. Dr. Collipp's own studies show that children should see the doctor on a one-to-one basis and then join a group of from ten to fifteen other overweight youngsters. The group helps shy fat children open up and encourages them to exercise more.

10. Young children need much parental help, the doctor finds, but teenagers need exactly the opposite. Teens are independent and the key to helping them change their eating behavior is to give them total responsibility for it. "Parents are out of it," says Dr. Collipp. "I tell teens that what they eat is up to them."

The doctor has some interesting advice for parents. He stresses that parents should *never* give children food to quiet them in the supermarket. Shopping snacks are powerful reinforcers of negative eating behavior. He also suggests, for the same reason, that the entire family refrain from eating while watching television.

CAUTION! GUILT AHEAD. Under no circumstances should you feel terminal guilt if you have given your child food rewards. Haven't all parents? Both overweight and thin children have received a food treat for having been good so that *in itself* is not the cause of obesity, just a practice to avoid.

Most pediatricians stress the need for the child's cooperation before diet treatment can begin. This is especially necessary for adolescents. "For some teenagers," says Dr. S.L. Hammar of Kaui-keolani Children's Hospital, "we must seriously question whether we do more harm than good by pressuring them to lose weight. Often, our best intended efforts and concerns only intensify the teenager's feelings of anger and rejection and make him feel more unacceptable."

According to Dr. Hammar, this negative reaction is especially prevalent when the doctor "considers obesity as a moral problem rather than a chronic disease." Such attitudes, he says, are readily perceived by adolescents and tend to drive them away from professional help.

It appears that in the case of children Dr. Right should be Dr. Super-Right.

The rebellious, confused overweight young person might benefit from psychiatric help if he or she is willing, usually in a group of other young overweights which has a nonthreatening title such as "Students Who Are Having Trouble With Their Health."

If you consider emotional assistance for your teenage youngster, here is the result of a National Institute of Mental Health study on the psychiatric treatment of overweight youth. You can use this as a guideline when evaluating a mental health professional.

A physician who is treating a child or adolescent must remember that as sensitive as the average child or adolescent may be, obesity usually carries with it heightened sensitivity. Such children often feel rejected, have a poor opinion of themselves and are depressed. It is a tragic irony that the very defense (fat) that a person erects against damage to his self-esteem is the stimulus for scoffing, derogatory attacks, humiliation and expressions of disgust by those one is trying to defend against. Love, understanding, compassion and support from even one person could lead a human being out from a lifetime of 'solitary confinement.' These young patients, who have always lived very much by themselves due to the ridicule and contempt encountered in school and other social relationships, have had very little opportunity to compare and check the validity of their dreams of glory, their goals and philosophy of life with other adolescents. The physician who is able to appreciate this sense of alienation from others and affords them the opportunity to examine their feelings and attitudes in the many situations of everyday living may be the first to provide them such an experience. An invaluable service which the family practitioner can offer to his fat patients is to help them differentiate between possible achievements and fantasized expectations. Thus, he can reduce the sense of frustration or failure experienced at their inability to achieve the impossible.

I have quoted at length here because this study's recommendations to psychological professions contain good information for parents as well. The trick to helping your overweight child seems to be in getting the right help at the right time. Perhaps that's not as difficult as it sounds since, as we become more tuned in to our own holistic natures, we are capable of listening more closely to what our children are really telling us.

Diet Fads Young People Should Avoid and the Secret of Youthful Diet Success

Helping pre-teens diet, as we have seen, is usually a matter of parental control. Not so with older children. With teenagers, before the problem of good diet can be approached, a great many bad dieting practices must be unlearned.

Fad diets are a parent's primary concern with adolescent dieting, as they can do more harm to health than losing weight can do good. We have only to remember the deadly macrobiotic diets of the 1960s. More recently a new and perhaps even more serious dieting craze has swept high school and college campuses. Increasing numbers of young women who want to be thinner in a hurry are being caught in a physically and psychologically damaging cycle of starvation, binge eating and punishing purges. Two Cornell University psychologists have named this practice *bulimarexia* and claim it is fast becoming widespread. One off-the-cuff estimate claims that as many as 25 percent of young women have tried this frightening solution to overweight.

Why don't our schools teach these young people about good nutrition? Unfortunately, it's not all that easy. Nutrition expert Dr. Hilda S. White says nutritionists are hard-pressed to teach young people better habits because they:

Dote on fad foods and snacks
Ignore nutrition
Rebel against parents
Are almost totally indifferent to their own health.

It's true that better nutrition education in the schools is needed, but says White, "Forcing nutrition education on teenagers is as bad as trying to open their mouths and force down spinach and liver."

Dr. White believes that the most effective way is for industry to add essential nutrients to favorite foods. Parents of overweight youngsters could help by buying enriched foods for their children's home use.

Along with fad diets, there is another questionable practice (sometimes even advocated by doctors) you may want your child to avoid. Human Chorionic Gonadotrophin, or HCG for short, has been used on adults with doubtful success, but no recorded harm that I could find. This is not the case for young dieters. "It has the property of promoting excessive connective tissue growth," reports Ann Scott Beller in her book *Fat & Thin: A Natural History of Obesity*, "and could thus have an unfortunate effect on cartilage in the face, the earlobes, and the hands in adolescents who are still growing."

Here's some good news! Once your child decides to go on a weight-losing diet he or she has a success secret even you don't have. What is it? *Children have more will power than adults!* If you have any doubts about this claim think about to whom those Saturday morning advertisers are beaming their messages. Think of the impact your children have in your family. Young people have a lot of determination, as you probably know. And they are more tuned in to learning new things. They're accustomed to and expect to learn so that doctors, in particular, are able to reach them with information where parents and even teachers may make no headway. But most important of all, they have a short record, if any, of diet failure. It's as if they were writing on a clean slate. They are usually very optimistic when they start a diet and deserve to be so. Of course, another good reason for optimism is that they are still growing taller. Thirteen year old Timmy, at five foot one inch and 160 pounds was badly overweight. But Timmy gained four inches in height during the year he dieted, his height catching up with his weight before he reached his goal.

Interestingly, up to the age of twelve, both boys and girls do equally well in the diet sweepstakes. After that, boys generally do better. Why is that? Because they exercise more, a subject we'll deal with (again) right now.

Exercise for Your Overweight Child

Good nutrition and a solid, non-fad diet, important as they are, are not the miracle prescription for taking off your child's excess weight. Exercise may be. Dr. Jean Mayer, the former Harvard nutritionist, now President of Tufts University, conducted a study that showed fat adolescents actually consumed *fewer* calories than lean teens. But they exercised *far* less. Fat teenagers in the study managed to stay relatively immobile even when participating in active sports.

The type of exercise really doesn't matter very much, says Dr. Mayer, as long as there is *enough exercise for a long enough time*. The same results have been observed in youngsters as have been seen for adults. When obese children are placed in an exercise program with thin ones, the overweights lose twice as much body fat.

If you doubt that your overweight child grows less and less active the older he or she gets, take a look at the results of this experiment. Young overweight patients were asked to wear a pedometer to measure their movement. They were instructed to put it on first thing in the morning and take if off last thing at night. The findings were illuminating. Boys aged five to eleven years averaged seven miles a day, while girls averaged only slightly less at 6.6 miles a day. At this age they exercised equally. The picture changes radically with teenage boys and girls. Boys averaged 5.6 miles per day but girls had dropped to 3.1 miles, less than half their activity of earlier years. Reseachers believe this significantly lower activity for girls accounts for the reason that they tend to gain back more weight than boys when they stop dieting.

Dr. Collipp asks his young patients to write poems about how they feel about being fat. One child wrote the following which illustrates what inadequate activity can do to emotions:

Fat is fat, there is no cure
You sit and sit while you are bored
You sit there and sit there thinking of why you are fat
But then you know that fat is that.

Perhaps this effort won't win a literary prize, but it does express the spirit of what it's like for an inactive fat child, sitting around and hurting, feeling bored and depressed.

Dr. Felix Heald, who works with obese adolescents at the University of Maryland School of Medicine, says that kids eat not because they're hungry, but because they're bored. One way to kill boredom is to get children interested in testing themselves against the challenges of physical exercise.

Experts recommend overweight youngsters participate in exercise or sports at least an hour every weekday and three hours a day on weekends. Sound like too much? It won't be, if your child is motivated and participating in an activity in which he or she is interested and successful. The important thing for parents to remember, say all the people in the know, is to be liberal with praise for any increase in activity and, whenever possible, to join in.

So that you can know what young people's sports burn the most calories, you can check the game chart on page 195, even show it to your child. He or she may be happy to discover that a favorite sport is good for them, too. But it's not a good idea for you to push an exercise in which your youngster feels awkward or "gross," no matter how many calories it expends. "My mother insisted I take tap-dancing lessons," recalls one bitter teen, "and all the others called me 'Jiggly Janice' because my fat jumped up and down with each tap." Of course, your child may be thrilled at the thought of aerobic disco dancing as exercise. The point is that it should be a personal choice.

Fat kids tend to feel tense, dissatisfied, lonely and rejected, despite avid efforts to gain approval and be liked. Overeating, especially among young girls, is often not so much a response to appetite as a response to emotional tension. The *Canadian Journal of Public Health* reported the following results for a group of overweight children in an exercise program: Initial psychological tests showed that the subjects possessed higher than average intelligence, feelings of depression, high drive level, social sensitivity and chronic unresolved frustration hostility. After a five month exercise program they were seen to be less shy and more venturesome and uninhibited.

Eating for the overweight child is a tranquilizer. Paradoxically, an equally available tranquilizer is exercise. The exercise tranquilizer works much better for the fat child because it reduces the weight which causes the tension in the first place.

Young overweight people are often interested in this information, so don't hesitate to give it to your child. It is another thing, however, to get them to participate in physical activity. Lethargy is the "disease" symptom of fat. But even lethargy can be overcome. "I think the individual who becomes aware," says researcher Dr. Raymond J. McCall, "that lethargy is standing between him and something he wants may do something about it." Dozens of scientific studies repeat the same results: exercise is a mood elevator; and elevated moods equal less overeating.

How can you as a parent encourage your overweight child to exercise more? One obvious answer is to set an example. Start putting some of your own good intentions into practice. Swing into action. The obvious benefits you're getting will make exercise more attractive to the whole family, especially your child. Here are some other ideas.

1. *Help your child with his or her posture and walk.* Overweight children often have terrible posture. It's not the weight that's pulling them over, but the shame. Make a big point of your child's growth in height. Have a measuring place in your home where you place a mark every so often. Comment about how much taller he or she looks when they stand up straight to be measured. Play the beanbag game to improve both walk and posture. Place one on your head and one on the child's head and see who can keep it on the longest. Chances are the child will win. Once he or she begins to stand taller, self-respect is enhanced.

2. *Provide them with necessary equipment.* If your child evidences an interest in a sport or exercise buy the necessary equipment or at least as much as you can afford.

3. *Give your child privacy to exercise.* Fat children have been ridiculed so much they are ashamed of their bodies. Surely you can understand this. If they choose to do calisthenics at home, allow them the privacy they'll need not to be embarrassed and, of course, never allow brothers or sisters to make fun.

4. *Help your child to swim without embarrassment.* Most children love the water, but have been traumatized by cutting remarks. You can make it easier for your children by helping them choose a flattering bathing suit and, if necessary, allowing them to wear some kind of cover-up, such as a T-shirt, while they're swimming.

5. *Give your child family responsibility.* This suggestion has more to recommend it than just good parenting. You'll also be

helping your child exercise. Give him or her household chores that require exertion. This will add to the total calorie expenditure. Don't overdo it though.

6. *Encourage your child to join local team sports.* Little League and Bobbysox Softball plus soccer and an assortment of other teams are year-round activities in most every community. Everyone can play, no matter what their level of ability. It's fun and provides a child with the possibility of success, a possibility an overweight boy or girl desperately needs.

With all your best efforts some fat children are too defeated or rebellious to accept your help. If this is your problem, you may want to consider sending your child (if he or she is willing) to a special diet camp for children, a place where both exercising and eating habits can be changed constructively.

Should You Send Your Child to a Diet Camp?

Before your child becomes enmeshed in a cycle of diet and exercise failure, you may want to give him or her a chance to succeed in a group of peers, all of whom are overweight. Your child will feel no scorn and will not be treated as a "problem child" but as a child with a problem.

The tough exercise schedule coupled with low-calorie meals can mean a twenty to forty pound (even sixty pounds in one case) weight loss over the course of the seven week camp. Frankly, most children don't like it at first, but most change their minds when they begin to see results. One former camper lost thirty pounds one summer, then came back the next summer and lost twenty more. "At camp, everybody has a common cause," he says. "While you're there, you complain that they're working you too hard and that you'll never come back. But when you go home and your friends all say 'Wow, you look good,' that's real incentive!"

Although diet camps for kids have a good reputation generally, there are some dissenting voices you should hear. Dr. Samuel Ritvo, a child psychiatrist at Yale University objects to diet camping. "Camping should be a pleasant experience," he says. "The youngster should have fun and the interest should be all his own and not his parents. Otherwise, it may be a miserable way to spend a summer."

Dr. Lee Salk, the famous pediatrician and author, thinks that getting a lot of fat kids together doesn't cure the problem. In fact, he reasons, it may be a reason for perpetuating the problem. Everyone's obese, so it must be okay.

Other psychologists worry about a "rebound effect" from enforced treatment which could predispose the overweight child to avoid further attempts at weight loss altogether.

But just as many authorities have come down on the side of diet camping. "There's no real harm, except the cost," says Sidney Werkman, M.D., professor of psychiatry at the University of Colorado. "In fact, there are major values. These camps allow overweight boys and girls to come out of the woodwork, to express what they think about themselves and to recognize their problems."

On this issue, as with most controversies connected with obesity, the jury is still out. Nevertheless, you as a parent can ensure your child has a good experience if you both decide to give diet camps a try.

1. Help to have realistic expectations for success. If they are grossly overweight, they will not come home sylph thin, but they will come home with a great deal more knowledge about themselves and their weight problem plus an improved self-image. Ask the camp director how much weight the child can expect to lose.

2. If possible, visit the camp in advance. At the least, arrange to talk with other parents whose children have attended to see what their experiences have been.

3. The best camps have counselors who are formerly fat children. They are going to have more empathy for your child than young adults chosen for their svelte figures alone.

4. Activities should be well-planned and varied. If exercise is reliant on machines, it's an indication that the camp may be understaffed or, at the least, noncreative.

5. Menus, while low-calorie, should be varied. If the food is monotonous, no matter how good for them, children will not learn to reeducate their eating habits.

Sometimes a diet camp is the first place a fat child feels like a "real" person. One very overweight teen at a Weight Watchers camp was thrilled she could learn baton twirling. "At school," she says wistfully, "only thin girls are asked to join the baton class."

If you want more information, you can get a listing of *accredited* diet camps by writing the Association of Private Camps, 55 West 42nd Street, New York, New York 10036. Prices vary with camp and length of stay but will probably cost at least $2,000, depending also on how much paid travel is involved. If that sum doesn't fracture the family treasury, you now have another option for helping your overweight child.

Diet Clubs for Kids

Diet camps may be out of the financial question for your child, or he or she may need year-round help. Give some thought to introducing your boy or girl to a diet club, maybe your own. Most of the major diet organizations have made special arrangements for youngsters. TOPS has Tiny Tops and Teen Tops, and Overeaters Anonymous has teen groups. A TOPS official observes: "The kids begin coming with their mothers, but they stay because they no longer want to be the fattest kid in school."

The same diet group dynamics are at work for your child that are at work for you — competition, group support, reward recognition. But there's a plus factor with diet groups for children, especially teens. Studies show this is the age when group therapy of any kind works best. Fourteen-year-old Linda tells why she lost 32 pounds: "I felt such a responsibility. I knew I must really work hard to show people I could do it."

Sometimes a little child can lead you. Brian, who says the kids at school called him "Rhino Man" joined a diet group, his 60 pound success bringing his mother into the group after him. Not content, Brian then worked on his father who joined six months later and lost over 100 pounds. What happened to "Rhino Man?" "Now the kids call me Brian the Lion," the boy says happily.

Two Mothers Talk About Their Overweight Children and Their Own Feelings

Catherine, mid-forties and weighing more than two hundred pounds, talks to me in her well-appointed living room, her blond hair still vibrant with highlights, her peachy-cream complexion a perfect setting for her lovely features. She has five children, three of whom are overweight.

"Both of my parents were overweight," she begins, "but I adored them, especially my mother. I used to think it wasn't so bad to be fat since she was fat. I can see that same thinking in my daughters. There's always this nagging in the back of my mind that if I could do something about my weight, then maybe they could."

Catherine's voice, firm and confident when we started, begins to break under the burden of her feelings of responsibility. "Of

189

course, I feel bad about my girls — very bad — but at least the oldest one is doing all right. She's into a career and must stay well-groomed so she pretty well 'passes' for normal." Catherine stops a moment, unaware that she has used a term which once meant crossing the racial color barrier, a term that labels her daughter a member of a minority group.

"My youngest daughter has the grossest problem," she goes on, hugging her courage about her like a protective coat, expressing aloud feelings she's never owned to before. "I ache for her but I don't dare say a word. She's too resentful to discuss weight except when she wants clothes.

"The thing I find hard to cope with in this younger generation is that they won't wear girdles. When I was young and fat, at least I held it in, but today they let it all hang out — and *over*.

"My girls say I put too much emphasis on weight — that today, things are different. I don't see the difference. Boys still stay away and people are cruel. Nothing's changed. I know what my kids are feeling. I've been there." For a moment she pauses, then adds softly, "I'm still there."

Joan, at thirty-nine, has what most overweight people would give anything for — height. At five foot ten inches her 150 pounds is well-proportioned on her frame. "I want to lose another fifteen pounds," she says, smiling confidently, knowing I understand, "but it's hard to lose the last few pounds when you can 'get away with them.' "

She didn't gain weight (an extra sixty pounds) until after her second baby. "I just couldn't seem to control my eating," she recalls. She fought it alone for a decade, then joined Overeaters Anonymous. "I lost the weight and began taking my daughter Laurie to meetings with me. She didn't have a weight problem at that time and was incredibly bored.

"I wanted her to come with me because I could see she was eating compulsively. I knew it was only a matter of time before the weight started piling on. You know you can talk to kids, explain, but they don't listen.

"When Laurie was sixteen she gained 60 pounds in one year. It was terrible! That sudden change in her was hard for our whole family. My other children are thin — even underweight. One child became anorexic because she said she didn't want to be fat like her mother and sister. We all had to go for counseling. I'll never forget how amazed the therapist was at the *obsession* the entire family had for food.

"I felt responsible for that. When I lost my weight, I changed my cooking habits drastically. I guess I tried to force my family to eat my way. I shouldn't have made such a big issue.

"I was so happy when Laurie finally started going to OA meetings with me again, even though it was terribly sad to hear her get up and tell the group she had never been able to talk to others before."

Joan brightens after this, saying that her family is communicating more and that Laurie has found more happiness and self-confidence than she had ever known, more than during her earlier thin days. I came away feeling that mother and daughter, as they say at any new birth, were doing fine.

Two Dozen Ways You Can Help Your Overweight Child and Yourself

Helping an overweight youngster can be frustrating, as you well know, but these children must be helped lest the burden of obesity will surely carry over into adulthood where even more discrimination faces them. The obese young man or woman is likely to be turned down for enrollment in college in spite of good grades or intelligence. (A University of Minnesota study says fat children on the average are 8 to 10 I.Q. points smarter than skinny kids.) After school, the obese young man or woman, no matter how qualified, is likely to be turned down for good jobs or, once on the job, passed over for promotion.

Beyond all these good reasons, your help is needed because a child's pursuit of slimness carries important emotional rewards as well. Fat children see themselves as fat *first*, just as racial minorities have a heightened awareness of their own color. Fat children are passive, thinking of themselves as individuals to whom things are done — not as persons who do things. And sadly, they see themselves as rejected by their peers, whether they are or not.

You are on your child's side. If anyone understands the problems of obesity, you're that one. Haven't you suffered them all yourself? Of course you have, but your very knowledge can hinder your child's weight loss, instead of help, unless you know how and where best to apply it. Here's how:

1. Don't try to instruct, nag or bribe your child into dieting. If he or she is under ten years, you can create a dieting "food envi-

ronment" and maintain good control. If your child is a teen, every bit of research shows that adolescents who diet most successfully have parents who interfere the least. When excessive concern is shown, the teenager often counters with resistance. Unnecessary "I'll show you" eating only adds extra pounds.

2. Do find the right physician for your child and consult him or her regularly.

3. Don't sabotage diet efforts with unconscious negativism. For example, if you child has recently failed on a diet, but expresses a sincere desire to start again, encourage him or her just as if this were the first diet attempt.

4. Fad diets are definitely unsafe for growing children. They are poor, nutritionally speaking, and, even worse, they don't work, setting up the familiar failure cycle which only adds psychological problems to figure problems.

5. Don't overfeed your child during illness. Many children gain a considerable amount of weight after surgery or illness because of enforced inactivity and sugary indulgence.

6. Keep mealtimes peaceful. Never allow the entire conversation to be centered on the overweight child's diet. This can only cause a defiant resistance to dieting in any form.

7. Don't try to hide or lock up favorite foods. You will only encourage your child to outsmart you. And, believe me, he or she can. I often ate forbidden goodies right under my mother's nose without her ever being aware.

8. Have low-calorie, vitamin-rich snacks available based on what your child's doctor allows.

9. Try not to treat your overweight child differently than your other children. Overweight children already feel different enough.

10. Don't feel guilty because you are overweight, especially if you are doing your very best for your child. Even if your child, out of unhappiness, blames you, don't feel guilty. You have problems enough without being further handicapped by self-blame.

11. Help your child build an exercise program that is adequate, emotionally comfortable and challenging. If that sounds good to you, too, then join in yourself. Praise him or her for all physical activity, no matter how minor.

12. Lower weight-loss expectations for your child. Sometimes overweight children do not lose weight dramatically. Moderate losses that are not regained can often be maintained until height catches up with weight.

13. Allow your adolescent child to be independent in that he or she assumes responsibility for dieting and type of food intake.

14. It may not be a good idea to cajole your teenage daughter with the dazzling possibilities of boyfriends when she loses weight. Not only does this reinforce her "nothingness" now, but it may give rise to disturbing fantasies. For example, overweight teenage girls (and thin ones, too) have not had time to learn to deal with their own sexuality, so that the thought of being confronted with a boy-girl relationship may have disastrous consequences.

15. Find a group of other young people with weight problems or a diet camp if your child is willing. Support from peers can make all the difference.

16. Work toward proper meal planning. Provide a variety of foods in the proper amount so that dieting isn't boring.

17. Remember dieting children need extra emotional support in all areas of their lives. Encourage them at whatever they try to accomplish.

18. Gently but firmly eliminate eating in front of television.

19. It seems silly to say today but, NEVER use food as reward or punishment.

20. Clean out any "food traps" you have in your house such as cookie or candy jars. Also, remove the remains of last Christmas' frozen fruitcake from the freezer. (It's just as edible frozen. I know!)

21. Try never to give your child the impression that your love or approval hinges on his or her losing weight.

22. Don't reprove your child when he or she eats something not on the diet. Your child will already feel bad enough. (Just like you do.)

23. You're not the law. Don't go through your child's pockets for tell-tale candy wrappers or look for chocolate smudges on a blouse. You are responsible for what they eat at home. They are responsible for what they eat outside their home.

24. Always have *on hand* all the foods on your child's diet plan.

Teach your children to love themselves by loving them. Your super-sensitive overweight child is very sensitive to the nuances of emotions, perhaps far beyond their years. Because they are so body conscious, they need physical contact — a kiss, a spontaneous hug, a touch. Your genuine, loving emotion will be picked up by your children who, in turn, will be more able to express their own emotional needs more openly. You will both need this kind of affection and trust while you help each other with your common problem. With understanding and love and knowledge, you can help give your fat child a childhood worth remembering.

Holism and Your Overweight Child

One of the most significant ways you can help your child is by integrating your own mind, body and spirit into a unified whole. In reality, this integration sends your child the message, "You can count on me, because I'm here; I'm all here."

Aiding your child to solve a weight problem while you are solving yours teaches an invaluable lesson. The lesson? Problem solving, after all, is the very essence of living. It is a part of life that is inescapable from the first tentative step to the end of our days. We parents can show our children that problem solving — even when it comes to a baffling problem like overweight — is a skill that can be developed if we apply our whole selves to finding solutions. We can show our children that problems are solved when people are willing to apply effort, take initiative, act creatively, use self-reliance, and be respectful of themselves no matter how many times they suffer setbacks.

Above all else, you can teach your children by your behavior that they must become independent and learn to work things out for themselves with your support and love. Most of all, you can give your child praise for willingness to take on a weight problem. It takes courage as you well know.

Holism means being able to meet the challenges of living with *all* your resources. You can help your child (and in so doing help yourself) meet what may be the biggest challenge of his or her life. It won't be easy. It won't be easy for either of you. But if you give guilt-free, loving support all along, your child will know how much you care. And, believe me, that's a priority. Under those extra pounds, every fat child is crying, "Love me!"

Now turn to the final *Break Out of Your Fat Cell* chapter for a kit bag full of survival goodies to take with you on your determined march through a whole, thin, healthy life.

I will help my overweight child in these ways:

1. I will not think of myself as a parent with a problem child, but as a parent with a child who has a problem.

2. I will guide my child to a sense of his or her own worthiness.

3. I will let my child know in everyday ways that I think he or she is capable and skillful.

4. I will be a friend when my child needs a friend.

5. I will help my child build and maintain self-respect no matter what his or her size.

6. I will try to give my child the fortitude to endure unpleasantness.

7. I will show by my behavior that I think my child is *real* just as he or she is.

8. I will show that I believe in my child's self-sufficiency.

9. I will not feel guilty about my own weight problem or my child's since I am doing my very best, and that is all anyone has a right to expect.

Game and Activity Chart for Overweight Children

Game	Calories expended per hour
Ping pong	200
Soccer	650
Shuffleboard	250
Softball	350
Tennis	450
Volleyball	350
Bowling	270
Badminton	350
Basketball	800
Football	650
Activities	
Rowing (peak effort)	1,200
Skating	500
Skiing	450
Fencing	300
Motorcycling	150
Wrestling	800
Gymnastics	600
Swimming	750
Walking the dog	275
Bicycling (moderate)	325
Doing homework	120

A Fat Child's Garden of Curses

Temptation	Calories
Cola (8 ounces)	126
Popsicle	106
Big Mac	558
French Fries (10)	137
Kentucky Fried Chicken (4 ounces)	283
Chocolate candy (1 ounce)	130
Potato Chips (1 ounce)	158
Peanut brittle (2 ounces)	125
Coconut cookies (5)	390
Pecan brownies (2 ounces)	224
Ring Dings (2½ ounces)	366
Apple pie (4 ounces)	360
Frosted cereal (1 cup)	143
Fudgesicle	110
Buttered popcorn (1 cup)	143
Jelly donut	185
Animal cracker (each)	12
Oreo (each)	50
Fig Newton (each)	59
Pizza (1 med. piece)	153
Potato Chips (10)	114
Hot dog (roll and weiner with ketchup)	310
Oh Henry	264
Snicker	260
Baby Ruth (1 ounce)	137
Milk Duds (1 ounce)	111
Mr. Goodbar	326
Tootsie Roll (1 ounce)	115
Chili con carne (without beans ½ cup)	256
Hershey Bar (plain)	266

Chapter Thirteen

Your Holistic Survival Kit

"Until you try, you don't know what you can't do."
— Henry James

How many years have you been telling yourself, "I'm too fat to . . .?" Too many years. Promise yourself that from this day on you're not going to deny yourself the right to live fully. Opening up the wide world for you to live in has been the whole purpose of *Break Out of Your Fat Cell*.

Our thin chauvinistic society has been feeding you a lot of baloney about yourself. Along the way you got the idea that you couldn't enjoy the same things that thin people enjoy — nice clothes, a social life, respect. Somehow you got the idea that you had to *earn* all the things that other people have as a right. Don't you believe it another minute. You don't have to earn the right to live fully; you were born with that right and your present size has nothing whatever to do with it. Remember? You are not going to blame yourself for your weight problem, you are just going to do something about it. *Self-blame will immobilize you; self-responsibility will energize you.* You're an adult, and as such, you are responsible for your life. Responsibility, for you, will never be a duty but a daily pleasure.

Walking Thin

One of the first things you can do for the newly integrated you, the person who is using the full powers of mind, body and spirit in a lifestyle assault on obesity, is to stop walking like a fat person. It doesn't matter whether you've lost all your weight or have 100 pounds to go, walk like you owned the world. Don't allow your chest to sag with defeat, it only forces out your abdomen. Pull your shoulders back and tuck your buttocks in. Stand as tall and straight (and thin) as you can and you will feel better and look better. If you have trouble bringing this off in the beginning, hum a favorite tune to yourself. It will help to lift your spirits and give your attitude a positive tinge. The important thing is to get rid of any "hangdog" attitude that tells you and the world that you're sorry you're alive. You don't have to apologize for walking upright with love and respect for yourself. Shakespeare expressed it best when he said: "Self love is not so vile a sin as self-neglecting."

The Right Clothes for the New You (and Where to Find Them)

Make a vow today, *right now*, that you will never again neglect your appearance because you think you're too fat to merit new clothes. Man or woman, you are a beautiful human being and have a right to be well-groomed. It is true that big people are more visible in a crowd, so there are some general do's and don't's which you will want to observe as you improve your appearance.

1. Avoid clothing that's too warm if you're still overweight. We have our own padding.

2. Don't be afraid of horizontal stripes, but try to keep them underneath a jacket.

3. Don't buy anything too small. You have the right to be comfortable. I don't know who started the awful idea that overweights should buy clothes too small as an incentive to lose weight. (Whoever they are, they should be consigned to a Dante-like eternity of popping buttons and broken plastic zippers.) P.S. Never keep clothes that don't fit you *now* in your closet. Put away the too-big and too-small; otherwise you'll be tempted to wear them.

4. Do consider becoming prints. You may look great in a geometric design.

5. Don't wear too many layers of clothes until you are close to your weight goal. A dress or blouse (shirt) with a jacket or sweater over it is fine, but more than two pieces can add unnecessary bulk.

6. Do wear colorful clothes. Most overweights are frankly sick of black, brown and navy blue. If it looks good on you and you feel good in it, forget the old admonition to stick to dark colors.

7. Do wear pants if they're not too tight.

8. Avoid armless styles with the exception of at-home garments.

9. Don't wear clingy fabrics until your bulges all turn to curves.

10. Do buy a few good clothes of fine fabric and fit, like European women do, rather than many cheaper clothes.

There is a controversy among overweight women about the wearing of foundation garments other than brassieres. (Not too many of us can get away with the braless look.) Some large women, especially the younger ones, wouldn't consider the steady torture of a girdle, but you'll admit there are certain styles that look better when your curves are straightened out. Keep an open mind.

Along with the new wardrobe you deserve, you also have the right to a flattering hair style and good makeup. I'm sorry to say that once I had such a low regard for myself that I neglected both. Today, with a flattering up-to-date hair style and some lessons in the art of applying makeup, I can feel self-assured no matter what public appearance I might face. In the long run, it's really much cheaper to get the right makeup and learn to apply it than to "collect" jars and bottles of every newly advertised cosmetic. Sure it costs a few dollars, but you're worth it, and don't forget that.

Wouldn't you think that with over 22 million women wearing size 16 or over, many stores would stock larger sizes? If you think so, you're wrong. Although the situation continues to improve as overweights become more vocal about their needs, your best bet to acquire a variety of stylish, moderately-priced clothes that fit well still rests with stores that specialize in the larger figure. Although Lane Bryant, Roaman's and Bond's (for men) have stores throughout the country, mail order is the only way many overweights can shop for new clothes.

There is one caution you should observe in ordering from mail-order houses. Sizes from house to house can vary, therefore most overweights find it best to order one outfit only until they are sure the size they think they wear really fits them in a particular manufacturer's clothes.

Now, get started on building a more adequate wardrobe. Buy clothes that give your spirit a lift, clothes that not only fit your body, but clothes that fit your new lifestyle. If you don't already have a favorite store or mail-order firm, check the list on page 211. The important thing to remember is that you will be able to reduce your weight much better if you care about yourself in every possible way.

Picture Yourself:
Photographic Tricks to Make You Look Great in Prints

It is very difficult to find a photograph of me when I was very fat. The ones that do stare out of the album are inexplicably angry, a grim, determined expression pulling down the corners of my mouth. I look at them and see a stranger, not the real person I remember. I hated having my picture taken.

Most of the few available photos (almost as rare as authentic Lincoln photos) show me hiding behind someone else, holding my daughter in front of me or wearing an enormous tent-dress which I fervently prayed covered my more than 100 excess pounds.

Fat photos of me are not rare because none were taken. Some loving family member was always pointing a camera in my direction. Such pictures are rare because I always managed to get to the developer first and destroy all those (prints and negatives) that were unbearable. When I destroyed those "awful" pictures, somehow I was symbolically destroying that fat girl in them.

Oh, how I wish I had known some tricks which would have made me feel more comfortable in front of the camera, so that I would not now be faced with a family album in which I am almost "the woman who wasn't there."

None of us is ever totally pleased with pictures of ourselves. We're too self-critical, even when we're thin. But you'll want to look as picture-perfect as possible until you have a more slender, healthy body and feel less self-conscious in front of a camera. And why not? The next time you are caught by a prying lens, here are ten tricks for you to use. The camera may never lie, but you *can* outwit it.

1. Have the photographer move in close. Your head and shoulders represent only 15 percent of your weight.

2. Suggest the photographer be artistic and shoot through flowers or leaves to obscure anything below the waist.

3. Watch your position. To get rid of an excess chin, lean your body forward from the waist, turn slightly and lower your leading shoulder. Another flattering pose, especially for men, is to prop your elbows on a desk or lean against a chair.

4. Try flattering lighting. Pose by a window so that one half the face is in shadow. This gives the highlighted side of the face a more oval look. This was a favorite pose of the late 1800's when round faces were prevalent. The painter Rembrandt even used this technique on his hefty Holland burghers.

5. Women should wear a soft neckline; the very best is a chiffon scarf, the very worst a scoop neck which shows four or five inches below the neckline.

6. Makeup can take off pounds for the camera's eye. Use darker base makeup under your chin so it won't pick up highlights and then work in a darker base from the point of your cheekbone on down.

7. For photos wear darker clothes.

8. What hair style photographs your face thinner? Use a longer fluffier hair style. It tends to reduce the size of your face.

9. Don't hold your hands on your waist or let your arms hang at your side; they only tend to extend your waist. If you feel more comfortable with your hands on your hips, then hold your arms loosely to allow the light to show between arms and waist.

10. What if you're caught by an amateur photographer with an Instamatic and you have no time to prepare clothing, hairstyle or lighting? Do this. Don't stand flat on your two feet. Quickly shift all your weight on one back foot bringing the other foot forward. This immediately bends one knee and gives a more flowing line to the body.

"No matter what their size," says Ted Sirlin, master photographer and former President of the Professional Photographers of America, "weight is the number one concern of every person I photograph."

According to Sirlin, looking too fat is not only the concern of the subject, but the photographic problem on which professionals spend the most time: "Cameras do have a tendency to exaggerate heavy parts," he says, "so we use dozens of techniques (like the ones above) to overcome this." The gadget that helps professionals the most is called a vignetter which any amateur can acquire. A vignetter fades out part of the picture, softens arms and shoulders and fuzzes the background so that you will seem to fade into it. When you can't tell where you end and the background begins, you tend to look much thinner.

When you have achieved the body you desire as a result of all the things you are now doing for yourself, you will adore posing for the camera. Until then, you will feel more comfortable if you keep these ten posing tricks in mind.

Meeting an Old Friend You Haven't Seen for a Few Years (and a Few Pounds)

It's easy to say, "Just don't worry about it, dear," but that doesn't always stop the gut-gripping fear of facing the look in someone's eyes when they see you've gained weight. I have heard too many other overweights tell stories of staying home from the class reunion or crossing the street to avoid a dear friend (and I've done both myself) to believe that it can ever be easy. But there are ways to minimize the trauma and even make these meetings more pleasant. There may be a few awkward seconds, but a truly good friend will very quickly get past your size change to the memories you share. Just remember that you have only to cope with a very few seconds — and you can do that.

1. Try to understand your friend's (or relative's) reaction, without putting yourself down. Back in Chapter Five, we talked a good deal about body image and how threatening your change can be to other people. You may want to review this chapter before you confront the situation.

2. Don't *expect* upset. Do you have any idea how many times we psych ourselves down? We believe, "My friends will think I'm awful because I've gained weight," when in reality, they are probably not thinking that at all.

3. They have changed, too. While we're busy worrying about what they'll think about our weight gain, they are probably worried about what you'll think about their changes. *No one ever stays the same.* For that reason alone, don't place an invisible but very real line between yourself and others.

4. You know how much your life is now changing for the better. It's not always possible for others to see our inner changes in an instant, but you won't be with them long before they become aware that you are somehow different. They will sense that the center of you is more at peace. They will get a growing feeling that you have gained a new self-esteem wrapped in an attractive air of maturity. People like you who are fully using their body, mind and spirit are practically irresistible in an era when so many lives have no anchor.

As of right now, refuse any longer to accept the concept that others will not like you or sneer at you because of your size. Unless you do this sincerely, you will pass up many of life's opportunities, opportunities that give you added strength to carry on the holistic diet program which will give you the healthy body you want.

Questions You Never Dared Ask Your Spouse, Your Doctor or Even Ann Landers

As the author of *The Thin Book: 365 Daily Aids for Fat-Free, Guilt-Free, Binge-Free Living,* I have received many letters from overweights, often containing questions they're unable or unwilling to ask others. I have gone in search of answers because I think knowledge goes far toward breaking down the fear mechanism. Let me share both questions and answers with you:

Question: I've lost more than 150 pounds. Should I have plastic surgery to remove the excess skin that hangs around my abdomen?

Answer: Any elective surgery is up to the individual, but if you're asking me if it's right to consider such a step, my answer is an unqualified yes. You have undergone a massive weight loss, and it's simply not fair to end up with a body that will never return to its original natural shape. Plastic surgery can help in most cases.

Dr. Peter Mosienko, head of the plastic surgery unit at Baylor University, says that the most common operations on the formerly obese are operations to remove excess skin and fatty tissue across the abdomen, buttocks, thighs, breasts and upper arms with the surgical removal of excess abdominal material (called the "apron") most common.

One of the doctor's patients, a man who had lost 175 pounds, had a massive apron, reaching to his knees, which would never disappear with exercise or further weight loss. This apron weighed 30 pounds. After surgery, the man was so pleased with his new appearance that he had a further thigh and arm reduction which accounted for another 30 pounds of weight removal, totaling 60 pounds in all. "The plastic surgeon is like a tailor," explains Dr. Mosienko, "who reshapes the body suit after weight reduction."

If you're interested in knowing more, contact the American Association of Plastic Surgeons, Emory University Affiliated Hospital, Division of Plastic Surgery, 25 Prescott N.E., Atlanta, Georgia 30308.

Question: Sometimes I eat so much, I'm sick, but I'm afraid to tell my doctor since he might get so disgusted he wouldn't help me anymore. Why do I binge?

Answer: The first thing you should know is that you're not alone. I've binged too. And I've cried, too. Binge eating can be physically debilitating but, in my experience, the emotional after-effects are even worse. Like you, I often wondered why I did such an obviously self-destructive thing.

Recent research into binging behavior by Dr. Joyce D. Nash, a Stanford psychologist who specializes in consultant work for diet groups, illuminates the dark corners of binging.

Binge eating, even up to 20,000 calories, is what we do to block a stressful event. It turns our anger and anxiety inward because we can't face confronting these emotions. Researchers now know that binge eating is an inappropriate reaction to two kinds of stressful living events:

1. Interpersonal events — you discover you can't communicate or assert yourself with others in a situation.

2. Intrapersonal events — you have a time-management problem or a personal behavior change that disturbs you.

Binging, in effect, is a safety valve which helps reduce stress. It is a poor way of letting off pressure, but one which gives you momentary relief, until you can become more assertive (refer to Chapter Four). That is why assertiveness for overweights literally means pounds and pounds in any reducing program.

Although most overweights can remember binges where they ate food just a cut above garbage (stale crackers, frozen pies, sugar from the bowl, etc.), Dr. Nash in her Stanford University research found that most bingers are really picky eaters. Surprise! Bingers usually crave a particular high calorie food and it must be readily available. Here is the best reason I've heard for clearing your house of potential binge foods.

There are other characteristics of bingers and some possible solutions you may want to consider below:

1. Most binge eaters binge once a week or more. Binge eating tends to escalate with age. In other words, if you think you'll grow out of it as you get older and wiser, you won't. Start trying to stop now.

2. Bingers usually don't binge all day as many think, and as you might think yourself. Studies show that a binge usually lasts from 15 to 60 minutes. If you are about to binge, you know in advance you will have to abstain for one hour at the maximum. *You have the strength to stop anything for one hour.*

3. Binge eaters don't know why they binge. Fat people don't seem to be able to perceive the stimuli that trigger their behavior. If you keep an eating behavior diary (and if you don't, start one), always list the emotion that preceded a binge. In this way, you will gradually come to recognize what stressful situations trigger binge eating, so that you can keep your guard up. One caution: Don't just look for negative emotions and miss the possibility of the "celebration binge." I once threw myself into a binge because I had received an award which I obviously didn't feel good enough about myself to think I deserved.

4. Binging is not a mindless thing. Psychologists were surprised to discover that we know what we're doing while we're doing it. We don't even feel too bad during the binge itself. It is after we gobble down a dozen candy bars that we become depressed, angry and hate ourselves.

An obvious solution to much binging is to stop putting too much pressure on ourselves and get to know what's going on in our heads and in our environment. And here's another helpful, if not surprising, tip. Dr. Nash follows a unique plan called, "prescribe the symptom." Here's how it works. Suppose you've binged on ice cream, eaten the whole quart (or half-gallon, for that matter). You can safely assume that ice cream is a binge food for you. Now work ice cream into your diet on a regular basis. For example, you can schedule one-half cup, or one scoop, for after dinner every night. Now the trick is that *you must eat it whether or not you want it.* When it comes time for you to eat it and you don't want it, you will discover that you can eat it without being out of control. You are finally in control of your binge food; it is no longer in control of you!

Question: I've lost weight before, but I can't keep it off. How can I maintain my weight loss?

Answer: You've just put your finger on "the name of the game" — maintenance. Many of us can lose weight; it's keeping it off that proves to be harder. Recognizing this, most of the diet clubs now have separate maintenance plans, even separate meetings for maintainers. (I wondered at this, until I discovered that the problems of maintainers can scare a still-losing dieter to death. Many of them think they won't have any problems once they lose their weight and are devastated to learn they will.)

The best ways I know to maintain weight loss are:

1. Add back foods one at a time so you can *know* (instead of guess) what they do to your weight. Too many times we try to return to pre-diet eating all at once and experience a terrifying weight gain, which for some of us just continues escalating. If, for example, you want to add back a potato, try adding a small potato three times a week to your regular weight-losing diet. If you continue to lose, then add another fruit per day or whatever food you want in your diet most. The idea is to give yourself a week between add-backs so that you can watch the scale to see just what this food does to your body.

2. Another good way to keep your weight down and fairly constant is to use this equation:

12 calories per pound of body weight (15 for men) times your ideal body weight equals weight maintenance. If you are a woman who wants to weigh 115 pounds, your equation would look like this:

$$115 \times 12 = 1,380.$$

In other words, you should limit your daily calories to 1,380. If you are a man whose ideal weight is 160 pounds, your equation would look like this:

$$160 \times 15 = 2,400.$$

You should limit your calorie intake every day to 2,400.

These calorie counts are for moderately active people. If you exercise regularly, you can add the calorie energy from the charts in Chapter Eleven to your daily intake.

3. Install an alarm buzzer in your "mental" scale to go off every time you show a gain of more than three pounds.

Question: I heard my doctor tell his nurse to put me in a placebo control. What does that mean?

Answer: A placebo is a pill containing no medicine. They are often called "sugar" pills, although I wouldn't think a diet doctor would think in such terms. Your doctor is probably making a study of a diet medication. He is probably using the group to which you were assigned to test how well people do with no real medication, when they think they're getting some. (Don't feel cheated. Research shows placebos work as well as most diet pills.)

Question: How can I possibly diet while I'm on vacation?

Answer: How can you possibly take a vacation from the things you are doing to change your life? Here are some dieters' vacation tips:

1. Don't drive way past your mealtime looking for the perfect restaurant. When I've done that, I've been ready to devour the placemat before the salad comes. Like a good soldier, you should carry emergency rations in the car. A thermos full of diet cola is my mainstay between stops.

2. You've seen the Fly Now, Pay Later advertising campaigns. You can also Fly Now, Diet Later. When you order your flight ticket, request their low-calorie meal and then try to sleep through the macadamia nut snacks.

3. Avoid an American-plan hotel because you will want to pick your own foods.

Question: I've got calorie counters and carbohydrate gram counters and nutrition books. Is there an easier way to get all this information?

Answer: Yes. The best, most inclusive, book that lists calories and all other nutriments for 2,483 different foods, from abalone to zwieback, is *Composition of Foods* published by the U.S. Government. If you want a copy, write to the Superintendent of Documents, U.S. Government Printing Office, Washington, D.C. 20402.

Question: I'm a night eater. Isn't that the toughest time to stay on a diet?

Answer: Night eaters have it tough, all right, but not as tough as afternoon eaters. The worst time of the day to stay on a diet is between three and six o'clock in the afternoon, according to a Diet Workshop study. The solution is to stay busy and interested. Most of us overweights overeat because we're bored and anxious, but we're less likely to eat when we are involved in absorbing work.

Question: I'm such an emotional person. What are the principals of weight-reducing which help to minimize problems?

Answer: This is a good question for which every overweight ought to have the answer, regardless of whether or not they think themselves emotional. Dr. Floyd K. Garetz, a psychologist at the University of Minnesota Medical School, recently compiled just such a list of principles which he calls the socio-psychological components of a good reducing plan. Here they are:

1. Try counter denial — We overweights often forget or miscount calories. Diets that make it more difficult for you to deceive yourself about the number of calories you've eaten are best. Eating plans which restrict the kinds of food you eat are one answer, since it is much more difficult for you to deceive yourself about eating candy if it is forbidden than it is for you to deceive yourself about how many calories of candy you have eaten.

2. Use rituals — Mankind has, throughout its history, used rituals to calm anxiety. Dieting is no different. Diet groups that have more or less complex or lengthy food preparation directions or diets that involve a good deal of preparation can answer this need for ritual. Diet plans that are billed as "easy to follow" may not be fulfilling this very necessary ingredient of the psyche.

3. Have self-esteem and pride in your body — You know what pain and a sense of failure your destroyed self-image has brought you. It stands to reason that an important factor in diet success would be to reverse this process and establish a sense of body

awareness which could reduce any mental anxiety due to loss of personal size.

4. Maximize your oral gratification — Obviously we overweights eat beyond nutritional needs because we experience pleasure in the form of oral gratification. Diets that require eating slowly and include plenty of chewy foods increase your pleasure without increasing calories.

5. Get the emotional support of a group — As Chapter Ten shows, joining a group which offers emotional support, a social outlet and acts as a censor to overeating can help make dieting less lonely and difficult.

6. Find the "magic factor" — When you follow reducing methods advocated by famous people or groups, you unconsciously invoke a magical component because of your deep need to have a powerful unseen ally. The early use of so-called "water pills" which promotes a rapid weight loss (diuresis) can often be seen as another aspect of the magic component.

7. Reduce temptation — This one needs no explanation. As subject to cravings and binges as we are, the more we are able to create a slender, food-controlled environment the better our chances at diet success.

8. Increase your self-control — "The Drinking Man's Diet" or any plan that allows alcohol tends to make staying on a diet more difficult. If you feel that you're sensitive to carbohydrates, especially refined sugar and flour, eliminating these can increase dietary control.

Your Wellness Inventory

The new concept of holistic medicine is one that defines our physical state by how well we are instead of how sick we are. It is a most positive, hopeful way for us overweights to look at our problem, too. By concentrating on our predominant wellness, we can then take the few health areas we need to work on and aim at them as if at a bullseye. Don't you think that focusing on how well you are puts the state of your health into a more logical perspective?

At this point, you may think you know what wellness means, but it has a special meaning in holistic medicine. What is meant by wellness? Most of us think in terms of illness and assume that the absence of disease indicates we are well. This is not altogether true. There are degrees of wellness just as there are degrees of sickness. The ultimate idea of wellness is to help you reach ever higher levels of being and feeling fantastic!

The first thing you need to do is to determine your own current state of wellness so that you can get an idea of where you are and where you need to go in your self-healing process. The best way I know of doing this is to take the Wellness Inventory offered by the Wellness Resource Center in California.

A sample of the questions you will be answering are on pages 212 and 213. From these you will get an idea of how comprehensive the 103-question inventory truly is. It costs just fifty cents and is worth many times that much to you.

The Whole You

This book has been a kind of journey, one which, I hope, has provided you with positive signposts all along the way. No one can force you to travel the road to your own integration. You are free to enter it or leave it at any point, but to deny it altogether leads to exquisite unhappiness. Ernest Hemingway once told a group of school children that the hell of life was you could leave it any time, but the idea was to go on and on and not quit until you had experienced it to the fullest. Another philosopher added her intuition of what Hemingway meant by "fullest," when she said, "Life's greatest achievement is the continual remaking of yourself so that at last you know how to live."

At last, you know how to live. You can free yourself from your fat cell, which is the prison of your guilt for being fat. Guilt is one of the most powerful emotions, and people will do anything to relieve it. In the past you and I have overeaten to relieve it. In the past you and I have punished ourselves for the crime of being fat. Sometimes if we have lost weight, we have done something to make sure we failed again. It becomes, after years of anguish, the only way we could live with the "wickedness" of being fat. No more!

But the secret of living, whatever your size, is to begin to believe the message that you are a complete human being. You are a complete being today. You are a complete being NOW. You will be healthier when you have lost weight. You will be able to accomplish some physical activities better. You will probably live longer. And you will be, without a doubt, happier. All this is true, but you don't have to wait until you are slender to become a complete human being. *You are that as you read this.*

I hope this book has helped you to learn this marvelous, thinning process of being whole by putting your mind, body and spirit to work for you. And I hope that you have come to believe that a full and dignified life is your right. As you begin to assert your human rights, you may risk, at first, not being liked, but if you don't allow yourself to take this small risk, you will cower in your fat cell forever, taking the blows of a thin, chauvinistic society and believing you deserve them. It is only when you risk asserting your rights that you can know true acceptance.

You are in charge, totally in control, from this moment on. Nobody else can live your life the way you can live it, or do it better than you can. There is no limit to what you can do.

The barred doors of your fat cell are swinging open. You are free.

▐||||| ◼ ◻ |

Where to Find the Right Clothes for You

Retail Stores and Mail-order

Lane Bryant, 2300 Southeastern Avenue, Indianapolis, Indiana 46201

Roaman's, Saddle Brook, New Jersey 07662

Sears Roebuck, Sears Tower, Chicago, Illinois 60684

Montgomery Ward, 600 West Erie, Chicago, Illinois 60607

Lana Lobell, Hanover, Pennsylvania 17331

Bellas Hess, Inc., Kansas City, Missouri 64116

The King Size Company (Men only), Brockton, Massachusetts 02402

Outsize Manshops (Men only) Mail Order Department, 86 Prospect Street, Hull HU2 8PG England

Nancy Austin Fashions, 2800 Las Vegas Boulevard South, Las Vegas, Nevada 89109

National Wholesale Company, Inc., Lexington, North Caroline 27292

▐||||| ◼ ◻ |

A Kit Full of Diet Survival Proverbs – Chapter and Verse

1. Don't continually test your willpower. If you had a lot, you wouldn't be reading this.

2. Stop playing the postponement game: don't postpone dieting, loving or living.

3. Take all the help you can get.

4. You don't have to solve your entire life problem today. Just take dieting a day at a time.

5. Be kind to yourself. Perfectionists are impossible to live with.

6. Having fun is essential to emotional health.

7. You have the power to change your life.

8. Falling down from a diet is not failure. Staying down is.

9. Don't worry too much about the adjustments others have to make because of your body change.

211

10. You have a right to the happiness your new body will bring you.

11. Three rules of successful dieting: Never get too bored. Never get too tired. Never get too hungry.

12. Don't allow one wayward bite to wipe out a diet. You don't deserve that much punishment.

13. Whatever it is, do it *now*!

14. Don't concentrate on the food you are giving up, but on the new life you are getting.

15. Talk to yourself of health, happiness and opportunity. Talk of victory.

16. Dare to reach deep inside of yourself. You will find something wonderful.

17. What people do or say against you has no meaning unless you agree with them.

18. You can erase undesirable eating behavior by simply not responding to it.

19. The more you live your life as you feel you should, the better you will think of yourself.

20. Choose success today.

21. Try *some* activity.

22. Stop talking about being depressed.

23. Always have on hand the foods your diet calls for.

24. You don't need negative people.

25. Make each day an emotional success.

26. Get rid of your "pound of flesh" this week.

27. The whole life is a statement of self-love.

28. The consistent dieter has a real contentment.

29. It is not what happens to you that creates problems, but how you react.

30. Strive for unity of mind, body and spirit. Unity's other name is self-confidence.

Wellness Inventory Sampler

Productivity, Relaxation, Sleep

04 ☐ If I am awakened, it is usually easy for me to go to sleep again.

09 ☐ I meditate or center myself for 15 to 20 minutes at least once each day.

Personal Care and Home Safety

12 ☐ I regularly use dental floss and a soft toothbrush.

17 ☐ I minimize my exposure to sprays, chemical fumes or exhaust gases.

Nutritional Awareness

20 ☐ I eat at least one uncooked fruit or vegetable each day.

29 ☐ I have a good appetite and maintain a weight within 15 percent of my ideal.

Environmental Awareness

30 ☐ I use public transportation or car pools when possible.

33 ☐ I set my thermostat at 60° or lower in winter.

Physical Activity

43 ☐ I jog at least one mile twice a week (or equivalent aerobic exercise).

48 ☐ I do yoga or some form of stretching-limbering exercise for 15 to 20 minutes at least twice per week.

Emotional Maturity and Expression of Feelings

51 ☐ I think it is OK to feel angry, afraid, joyful or sad.

53 ☐ I am able to say "no" to people without feeling guilty.

Community Involvement

65 ☐ I would at least call the police if I saw a crime being committed.

68 ☐ If I saw a car with faulty lights, leaking gasoline or another dangerous condition. I would attempt to inform the driver.

Creativity, Self-expression

77 ☐ I like myself and look forward to the future.

79 ☐ I find it easy to express concern, love and warmth to those I care about.

Automobile Safety (optional)

81 ☐ I wear a lap safety belt at least 90 percent of the time that I ride in a car.

84 ☐ I frequently inspect my automobile tires, lights, etc., and have my car serviced regularly.

Parenting (optional)

94 ☐ I do not store cleaning products under the sink or in unlocked cabinets where a child could reach them.

98 ☐ I frequently touch or hold my children.

Reprinted with permission from the *Wellness Workbook for Health Professionals,* copyright 1977, John W. Travis, M.D., published by the Wellness Resource Center, 42 Miller Avenue, Mill Valley, California 94941.

HOLISTIC LIFESTYLE CHANGE 13

For the rest of my life, I will try to:

1. Give myself more real pleasure than food punishment.

2. Be self-respectful.

3. Never postpone living because of my size.

4. Never participate in my own humiliation.

5. Accept total responsibility for my health, but never guilt for having been fat.

6. Attain my highest level of wellness — physically, emotionally and spiritually.

About the Author

Jeane Eddy Westin has a unique perspective when she writes of the problems of overweight in her books and in more than 250 magazine and newspaper articles. Having lost more than 100 pounds herself she couples an insider's understanding with the investigative eye of the trained journalist. As a result, her most recent effort, *The Thin Book,* has become a supportive, optimistic handbook for a legion of dieters.

She teaches college writing courses, conducts body image/sex workshops for the overweight and has been a featured speaker on many subjects for colleges and professional organizations.

Among her affiliations are The Authors Guild and the American Society of Journalists and Authors. She is listed in *Who's Who of American Women, Contemporary Authors* and *Working Press of the Nation.*

She lives with her husband and their daughter in Sacramento, California.

Select Bibliography

Beller, Anne Scott, *Fat & Thin: A Natural History of Obesity*, McGraw-Hill, New York, 1978.

Bruch, Hilde, M.D., *The Importance of Overweight*, W.W. Norton & Co., Inc., New York, 1957.

Coleman, Emily and Edwards, Betty, *Body Liberation*, J.P. Tarcher, Inc., Los Angeles, 1977.

Edelstein, Barbara, M.D., *The Woman Doctor's Diet for Women*, Prentice-Hall, New York, 1978.

Eden, Alvin N., M.D. and Heilman, Joan Rattner, *Growing Up Thin*, Berkley, New York, 1975.

Farquhar, John W., M.D., *The American Way of Life Need Not Be Hazardous to Your Health*, Stanford Alumni Association, California, 1978.

Grosswirth, Marvin, *Fat Pride: A Survival Handbook*, Jarrow Press, New York 1971.

Huxley, Laura Archera, *You Are Not The Target*, Wilshire Books, California, 1963.

Rubin, Theodore Isaac, M.D., *Alive and Fat and Thinning in America*, Coward, McCann & Geoghegan, New York, 1978.

Stuart, Richard B., M.D., *Act Thin, Stay Thin*, W.W. Norton, Inc., New York, 1978.

Westin, Jeane Eddy, *The Thin Book: 365 Daily Aids for Fat-free, Guilt-free, Binge-free Living*, CompCare Publications, Minneapolis, Minnesota, 1978.

Yudkin, John, M.D., *Sweet and Dangerous*, Peter H. Wyden, Inc., New York, 1972.

Index

School of Medicine, 23, 34
University of Colorado, 188
University of Illinois, 23
University of Louisville, 23
University of Maryland School of
    Medicine, 185
University of Miami, 24
University of Minnesota, 117

W

Wachtel, Kenneth, 93, 94
Walking, 162, 163, 197
Washington, George, 11
Weight loss
  becoming comfortable with changes
        due to, 124
  personality changes due to, 139
Weight problems
  understanding your, 15-27
Weight Watchers, 145, 146
Weinberg, Dr. Abraham, 2
Wellness inventory, 208
  sampler, 212, 213
Wellness Resource Center in
    California, 209
Werkman, Sidney, M.D., 188
Wertmuller, Lina, 104
White, Dr. Hilda S., 182, 183
Wirtshafter, David, 23
Woman Doctor's Diet Book for Women,
    91, 163

Y

Yale University, 187
You Are Not the Target, 103
You Can Be Your Own Sex Therapist,
    102
Yo-Yo syndrome, 20
Yudkin, Dr. John, 33, 34, 36, 37

Z

Zorba the Greek, 79

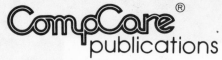

CompCare® publications

A Division of the Comprehensive Care Corporation
Post Office Box 27777, Minneapolis, Minnesota 55427

for faster service on charge orders
call us toll free at:

800/328-3330

In Minnesota, call collect 612/559-4800

ORDER FORM

Date _____

Order Number	Customer Number	Customer P.O.	☐ ☐ ☐ ☐ ☐ 1 2 3 4 5	For Office Use Only

| UPS
1
☐ | PP
2
☐ | PPD
3
☐ | PPD
CHGS
4
☐ | WILL
CALL
5
☐ | OUR
TRUCK
6
☐ | CARRIER |

BILL ORDER TO:

Name _____

Address _____

City/State/Zip _____

Non-profit organization, please show tax exemption number [_____]

Signature _____ Sales and use tax number _____

SHIP ORDER TO: (If other than above)

Name _____

Address _____

City/State/Zip _____

Telephone _____ Purchase Order (if required) _____

☐ Please ship back-ordered items as soon as possible

☐ Please cancel order for items out of stock

(Catalog number 03095)

☐ Please send _____ copies of *Break Out of Your Fat Cell . . . at $5.95 each.*

☐ Please send me the CompCare Catalog of more books and materials for growth-centered living. (No charge.)

PLEASE FILL IN BELOW FOR CHARGE ORDERS
Or enclose check for total amount of order.

Prices subject to change without notice.

Account No. (12 or more digits) from your credit card

[☐☐☐☐☐☐☐☐☐☐☐☐☐☐]

Check one

☐ VISA   ☐ MASTER CHARGE   [☐☐☐☐] Master Charge—also enter 4 digits below your account no

Your Card
Issuing Bank _____   Expiration Date of Card _____

Credit Card
Signature _____

TOTAL PRICE _____

4% Sales Tax _____
(Minnesota residents only)

Postage & Handling charge _____
Add .75 cents to orders totaling less than $15.00
Add 5% to orders totaling $15.00 or more

GRAND TOTAL _____
(U.S. dollars)

All orders shipped outside continental
U.S.A. will be billed actual shipping costs.

VISA®   **master charge** THE INTERBANK CARD

Date Due